OVERCOMING

THE

ODDS

Antonio J. Webb, M.D.

Printed in the United States of America
First Printing, 2014

ISBN-13: 978-0-9909833-0-9 (p)
ISBN-10: 0-9909833-0-7 (p)
ISBN-10: 0990983315 (e)
ISBN-13: 978-0-9909833-1-6 (e)
LCN: 2014920436

For autographed copies or bulk orders, please visit:
www.antoniowebbmd.com

I dedicate this book to my youngest brother, Jonathan Immanuel Webb, who passed away after a battle with Leukemia in 2008.

Until we meet again.

Sunrise: 28 June 1986
Sunset: 8 Dec 2008

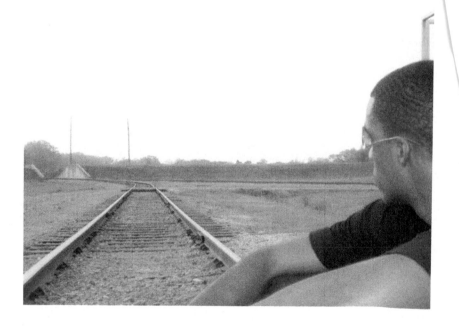

CONTENTS

PREFACE

I wrote this book to inspire those who may think the only way out is by turning to the streets, selling or using drugs, or relying on gangs to get them through life. I also wanted to let others know that if I achieved my goals, despite being faced with seemingly insurmountable odds, they can as well.

Whether you are forty years old in the middle of your career, or a sixteen-year-old high school student with dreams to become an engineer, this book is for you. It is divided into three sections. Each section voices the trials and tribulations I faced and was forced to overcome during my childhood, military career, and path to medical school. In addition, after each chapter, you will find practical advice on how to face life's challenges head on.

I hope that as you read through the upcoming chapters, you will be able to utilize the advice given as guidance, when you are met with obstacles in life or faced with the challenge of *"Overcoming the Odds."*

SECTION I:
CHILDHOOD

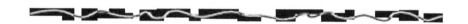

INTRODUCTION

According to the International Center for Prison Studies, the United States has the highest percentage of prisoners in the world, at 716 prisoners per 100,000 people. While blacks make up only 30 percent of the US population, they account for an astonishing 60 percent of those imprisoned. Louisiana has a higher rate of imprisonment than any other state in the US, followed by Mississippi, Alabama, Oklahoma, and Texas. When compared to other countries, Louisiana's incarceration rate is nearly 5 times Iran's, 13 times China's, and 20 times Germany's.

It is said that one in three black men can expect to go to prison at sometime in their lifetime. The incarceration rate is so high that young black men without a high school diploma are more likely to go to jail than to find a job, thus perpetuating a cycle of poverty and crime. Within five years of release, about half of those who were incarcerated end up returning to prison.

In Louisiana, a two-time car burglar can get 24 years in prison without parole. A trio of drug convictions can land you at one of the top 10 worst prisons in America, such as the Louisiana State Penitentiary at Angola or the Orleans Parish prison in New Orleans – for the rest of your life.

My greatest fear, as I grew up in the dangerous poverty-stricken environment of Shreveport, Louisiana, was that I would become a statistic – just another black male who'd been incarcerated or sold and used drugs. Or even worse – just another body six feet under. I viewed each new day as a day closer to achieving my dreams, because failure was not an option.

A study in 2003 showed that Shreveport ranked number 12 as the most dangerous city in the country, only behind cities such as Detroit, Memphis, and New Orleans. The report used U.S. census definitions of metropolitan statistical areas and tallied its rankings based on 2003 FBI data kept in six categories: murder, rape, robbery, aggravated assault, burglary, and motor vehicle theft. In Shreveport, these crimes were an everyday occurrence while growing up.

In certain areas of Louisiana, groups of individuals wore specific colors to "represent" their gang affiliation. The Bloods could be seen wearing all red, while the Crips wore all blue. If, by chance, you wore the wrong colors and were caught at the wrong location, you could have gotten yourself in deep trouble. These individuals migrated in groups and were seldom found in places alone. It was for one's own good that you knew what parts of town belonged to what gangs, so to avoid wearing certain colors in those areas. In a neighborhood called Jacks Quarters, red was the color to wear. In the Westside of Queensborough, it was blue.

The reality of the situation hit me hard one gloomy Sunday evening while walking home from South Park Mall. I was with my cousin and brother, when a car drove up next to us.

"What's up man? It's Piru all day. What set you claim?"

I didn't know how to respond to that, so I just kept walking. Then, I glanced over and noticed a shiny object pointed in our direction as the guy in the car flashed his chrome handgun towards us. My heart skipped beats as my life flashed before my eyes. Barely managing to keep our cool, we just kept walking and hoped he would drive off. Luckily, after what felt like ages, the person with the gun realized we weren't who he was looking for and just drove off. We were just wearing the wrong colors at the wrong place, and at the wrong time.

Times like this seemed to happen quite frequently. Being around guns and individuals who had either been shot before or had "knocked off" several people seemed to be the norm.

One particular individual, who fell into the latter category, was known as Jet. Jet was a few years older than me and had been incarcerated several times for petty crimes. Word around town was that he had knocked off a few people.

Knocking people off earned you stripes in the hood, meaning that you were respected. Some people earned stripes by "hitting licks" which meant either robbing a person, place or stealing something of high value. Other people earned stripes by getting into multiple fights and beating up other individuals. And then some just earned their cred because they had been around for a while. Those people were referred to as "OG" or "G" (original gangster or gangster).

The last I heard, Jet was in prison doing hard time for a lick he had pulled.

And then, there was Jay.

Jay was highly regarded in the hood and in school because of his size. At 6'1 and 205 pounds in middle school, he demanded respect and respect was what he got. Together, we attended Hollywood Middle School, where our principal, Mr. Simon, was known for his flashy suits and his dreaded paddle spankings. Whenever someone acted up in school, they met with Mr. Simon for a personal meeting with the paddle.

One day, I was being my typical rebellious self and decided not to head to class when the bell rang. Instead, I decided to pick on one of my female classmates. She didn't take it very well. I ended up sitting in front of Mr. Simon, explaining myself, and begging for redemption. My plea for forgiveness did not work; I was paddled and I never picked on that girl again.

Mr. Simon had other, more clever, ways of disciplining us and keeping us in line. Fighting was always frowned upon, and Mr. Simon had a way to discourage it. Whenever two people felt the need to fight or solve a dispute, Mr. Simon had those individuals put on boxing gloves and duke it out in an old vacant classroom. If someone bullied another student, Mr. Simon would get the biggest person at our school, Jay, to fight that person. Needless to say, these boxing matches kept us in line and discouraged a lot of us from fighting.

Jay and I eventually went to different high schools. I played on the freshman basketball team at my school and he played football at his high school. He was very good at football and we all knew he would make it to the NFL, because of his size and speed. Several big college programs recruited him. He decided to attend Grambling State University, and that's where things started going downhill.

Word on the street was that he started messing with drugs and hitting licks to feed his habit. That landed him in and out of jail, only to repeat those same mistakes over and over again. I never saw him during that time, but our mutual friends stated that he had lost the majority of his weight from using drugs.

Hitting licks and using or selling drugs usually meant associating with the wrong people. Owing people money or hitting a lick on the wrong person meant someone would come after you. An OG once told me, "Always back your car in wherever you go. Angle it whenever you're in a long line so that you can easily get away, just in case someone ran up on you." The bad things Jay ended up doing eventually caught up with him years later.

From what I heard, Jay pulled up to a corner store to get gas. When he stepped out of his car, he was shot seven times. Due to his outstanding warrants, he was taken straight to jail but not before having surgery for his gunshot wounds. Several bullets injured his intestines and other organs, leaving him with a colostomy bag (drainage bag that allows you to defecate) and 10 years in prison.

In October 1998, a series of bank robberies occurred in Shreveport and its surrounding cities. Every few days, a new bank was hit. Armed men, wearing black ski masks and carrying large weapons, barged into banks and demanded large amounts of money. They continued to find and hit vulnerable spots for easy getaways, such as banks close to highways.

The Home Federal Savings and Loan bank, located on a popular street called Youree Drive, was the third bank robbed in nine days. Three armed suspects entered the empty bank, while a fourth suspect waited outside in a beige Cutlass Supreme car. One of the robbers fired shots inside the bank, but luckily no one was hurt. As they left the bank, witnesses saw the robbers tossing clothing from the car into a nearby dumpster.

The same car was later seen at the house of my friend, Marlo.

Marlo was my best friend's cousin and was known for getting a lot of chicks. He stood 5 feet 4 inches and was dark in complexion. These traits seemed to attract a lot of women back then. But, his charm and good looks couldn't keep him from getting caught.

Authorities ended up arresting Marlo, along with another one of my childhood friends, Little Fred. Some of the stolen money and a few weapons were recovered. Marlo and Little Fred each received a sentence of 10 years behind bars. We didn't hear much more about either of them after that incident, we just knew they had been locked up for a long time. And we accepted it. Because that's the way things happened in Shreveport.

It seemed like every few months, another one of our friends was getting locked up or killed. It wouldn't be long after that I would see my first dead body.

While driving to visit a friend one evening, I decided to stop by a corner store to get a drink. As I pulled up, I noticed that there were several people standing outside and looking at something on the ground. Curious, I joined them and saw a young black male lying motionless on the sidewalk. Blood was splattered everywhere, including on his brand new, white Nike tennis shoes. His body was covered with a white police drape and the area was blocked off by yellow police tape. I was taken by surprise as people walked around carelessly, as if nothing had happened. Apparently, he owed money to some drug dealers and after he didn't pay up, they came after him.

Then, there was Kurt.

Kurt belonged to a gang in Shreveport called the Lakeside Kings. He made the one mistake one should never make when in a gang – get caught by yourself. Rival gang members caught Kurt in the streets late one evening, without his fellow gang members, and gunned him down. His body was left to bleed to death in a dark alley behind a high school. Authorities never caught the person who shot him. As for myself, all I know was that one day I was speaking to him like any other, and the next day he was dead.

My closest friends and I lived in a neighborhood called Meadows and we called ourselves the Meadow Boys. We migrated in groups and would sometimes have squabbles with other rival neighborhood guys. We were known for pulling tricks around the neighborhood such as knocking really hard on people's doors and then running quickly to hide before they came to the door. We also attacked school buses as they came to drop off neighborhood kids. Sometimes, we skipped school to throw house parties when our parents left for work. Senior Skip Day became a yearly tradition where everyone bailed out on class and headed to party with the graduating seniors. Most years, it was held at a local park where we listened to music while sharing the latest gossip from around school.

One day, we decided to throw eggs at a bus filled with middle school students. The school we attended dismissed earlier than the younger kids, so we decided to gather the eggs and hide behind some bushes in the Meadows to wait for the bus. We waited and waited, until I peeped over the bushes and saw a big yellow bus heading towards us.

"Here it comes, here it comes," I yelled.

It was hot that day, so most of the windows on the bus were down. One by one, we threw a dozen eggs at the passing bus. We then ran back towards the bushes as we heard screams from the kids on the bus. Even though the bus driver stopped and yelled profane language at us, we thought it was fun to see the young kids scream as they got hit with eggs. We attacked the same bus several more times that year. However, when our parents gave us a hard time about eggs coming up missing, we transitioned to water guns instead. This eventually led to neighborhood water gun fights, followed by fistfights when the other kids got mad.

The Meadows was located close to an elementary school called Westwood. Nearby was a railroad track where we often threw rocks at the trains as they approached. Close to the railroad track was a basketball court, where I could be found almost anytime I wasn't studying.

One day, my cousin George lost his pager while playing basketball at Westwood. Understandably upset, he paged and paged it until someone finally returned his call.

"Hey man, I lost my pager. I need it back."

It turned out, a guy by the name of Tim found it and wouldn't agree to return it. My cousin was the type of person who would get upset about every little thing, and when someone did something to disrespect him or said something he did not like, he took matters into his own hands. I often rode with him, in his old white Ford LTD car, when he received calls to make drops. This placed me in the vulnerable situation of getting caught with drugs, but I didn't want to inconvenience him by having him take me home before making the drops. Whenever he got a call, we made drops to people around the city. The LTD didn't have a stereo, so we had a handheld radio player that we kept in the backseat. We listened to whatever was hot back then, probably Juvenile or Master P. I often sat up front and my job was to look out for "one time." We called the police "one time" because it only took one time of getting caught before you were going to jail. And you only looked once in their direction, as doing a double take might have attracted too much attention. Under George's seat was always a 9mm gun, which we stole from the neighbor's house one day while he was away. We needed it for protection. At least, that's what I always told myself.

Since George felt like Tim disrespected him, he decided to take matters into his own hands. One day, we found out that Tim was playing ball at the Westwood basketball court. We decided to pay him a visit.

We hopped into our friends' minivan and drove to the court. As we rode past, we saw several people playing aggressively on the basketball court, sweating from the hot summer heat. Without thinking twice, my cousin opened fire into the crowd of basketball players. One by one, they quickly dropped to the ground. I couldn't believe my eyes. The guy only took a pager, which had probably only cost $15-$20, and my cousin just tried to kill him. What I couldn't believe most was that I was a part of what just occurred and would be deemed an accessory to murder if anybody had been shot or killed. But, luckily, no one was injured and we never heard anything else about the shooting.

It was from that point that I knew my cousin wasn't someone to mess with. I also realized that I needed to watch who I associated or hung out with. Regardless, I continued to find myself around these individuals throughout my time in Louisiana, and eventually found myself getting into trouble right along with them.

…

"Stop right there!" yelled an older white gentleman with a deep country accent. It was like he had appeared from nowhere. I turned to my friend; both of us had startled looks on our faces. We just knew we would be going to jail that day. Though we had gotten away with it many times before, that was the day we wouldn't.

My friend and I made it a weekly habit to steal gas. Our prime locations were gas stations with pumps near open roads, so that we could steal the gas and speed away quickly without getting caught. We had done this several times before that day. I'm not sure if I was more scared of going to jail or having my dad find out. I knew if my dad did find out, my punishment would have been way worse than going to juvenile jail. Luckily, we didn't have to go to jail and were let go to our parents. Unfortunately, not every one of my family members was as lucky.

My little brother Jonathan was witty, intelligent, and a genius with computers. Whenever we had a problem with a computer, everyone knew who to go to. It was simple to him and came natural. We all knew he would make it big one day—and he did— too big and too fast.

ADVICE:

One simple mistake or arrest could cost you your entire career. I didn't realize how much of an impact an arrest would have on my career, until applying for medical school and filling out applications for jobs. I did, however, have to be truthful and answer "Yes" to the arrest history question. I even had to explain the arrest during my medical school interviews.

After applying and interviewing at a medical school in Arizona, I received a phone call from an unknown number one evening while at work. It was the doctor and interviewer from the medical school. He was passing through Texas and wanted to meet with me to discuss my application. I frantically called a good friend, who was already in medical school at the time, and told him what just happened. Did he want to tell me I was accepted in person? Why did he want to meet with me on New Year's Eve? I wondered. I agreed to meet with him and we met at a local gas station that had a Subway restaurant attached to it.

I nervously gathered my freshest suit and headed to meet the doctor. When I walked in, I could see that he had been waiting for some time. I was nervous and didn't know what to expect. The admissions board had met, discussed my file, and now he wanted to further discuss my arrest.

After 30 minutes of explaining myself, we ended the meeting.

Unfortunately, weeks later, I was sent a rejection letter. I personally believe the arrest cost me that medical school admission.

Most applications have a section that asks, "Have you ever been arrested?" "Have you ever been convicted of a felony, misdemeanor, or DWI?" Even if you have the appropriate degree, license, or certification and are fully qualified for the position, a mark on your record will haunt you for years to come. It may also end up costing you the job offer. Yes, there are lawyers who will charge you thousands of dollars to seal or expunge your record, however, government officials and other top-secret agencies can still see sealed records.

The best thing to do is to stay out of trouble in the first place. Use common sense. A lot of it has to do with being in the wrong place at the wrong time, and hanging around the wrong crowd. If you know your "so-called" friends are going out to do something illegal, don't go along. Yes, they may call you names. Yes, they may choose to not remain friends with you. But ask yourself, are they that good of a friend in the first place if they are allowing you to do something illegal?

If you have been convicted of a crime, answer truthfully. If you are caught lying, you may be excluded from consideration. If you are hired, and then your job finds out about your arrest, you may be terminated. A U.S. Department of Justice report showed that students who have been arrested, even for minor crimes, face extra obstacles in an already shaky job market. You will already be faced with an overwhelming amount of obstacles and challenges in the path of your career of choice; don't create extra obstacles that you will have to overcome.

What appears on a criminal background check:
- Basic identifying information such as your full name, date of birth, age, and driver's license number
- Any felonies or misdemeanors on your record
- Current and past arrests and court warrants
- Federal and state tax liens
- List of all known relatives
- Any property ownerships
- History of marriages or divorces

Potential reasons employers may choose not to hire you:

- Enforcement of employment laws: in order to avoid negligent recruitment charges, an employer may choose not to hire a convicted criminal as a potential candidate for the job
- Work place safety: some employers believe that hiring previously convicted individuals decreases the safety of their working environment
- Security: some jobs, such as the military, require a certain level of security clearance before hiring an individual. If you have a criminal record, you may not pass the employers security requirements

How to deal with employers after a criminal record:

- Be honest and upfront
- Express your remorse and identify what you have learned from the occurrence

A KNOCK ON THE DOOR

*B*ANG! BANG! BANG! The knocks on the door were followed by a loud, gravelly voice that echoed throughout the house.

"We have a warrant for Jonathan Webb! We need to search the house!"

It was 2:00 pm on a Wednesday afternoon when the busy street we lived on was suddenly flooded with cops and the FBI. They were equipped with enough weapons and armor to start a war. There were at least 5-10 cops who showed up that day, all with guns drawn. Some surrounded the house from the back while others entered through the front. They had come to look for my little brother and shut down the illegal computer operation he was running.

It turned out my brother's extravagant spending had garnered the attention of the FBI, and they had been watching him secretly for the past eight months. They parked unmarked cars across the street from our house and had been snapping photos to use as evidence.

...

"Let me drive your car to school today, I'll give you $100," Jonathan once stated to me.

Months later, he spent $8,500 on a new truck of his own. That didn't include the several thousand more dollars he spent painting it and placing expensive, spinning rims on it. By the time the FBI raided our house, they calculated that he had profited over $30,000. At the age of 16, that was a lot of money. So much money, in fact, that people began to plot ways to rob him. This led

15

me to have many heart to heart conversations with Jonathan about his behavior – I was desperately worried about him at the time.

Fortunately, since he was 16 and a minor, the cops let him go. Their main concern was that his illegal computer operation was shut down. But then, without any steady income to support the expensive spending habits he'd become accustomed to, he needed new ways to make more money.

It's a known fact that the people you hang around will have a large impact on the person you become. If you hang around drug dealers, chances are you will soon find yourself dealing drugs. If you hang around doctors and lawyers, you're likely to pursue those paths.

Before I realized it, Jonathan began to hang around individuals who were up to no good. One thing led to another and before long, I received a phone call notifying me that Jonathan had been arrested and was now in jail.

Jonathan and his group of friends had come up with a plan to steal money by robbing people at gunpoint who were coming out of ATMs – a quick way to get cash but also a quick way to end up in prison.

When I discovered that the person who'd actually had the gun was out on bail, I was infuriated. My family didn't have the bail money and we couldn't afford to get Jonathan out.

The unfortunate reality is, when you can't afford bail, you are forced to sit in jail until your court date – no matter how long that might be. My brother waited in prison for a *year* until his court date. I visited him whenever I could get to Louisiana from Texas, where I was living at the time.

And then came the verdict.

Juvenile life – five years in prison for armed robbery.

Jonathan was only 16 years old, with a felony, and a good portion of his life had been wasted.

During those five years, he moved between various institutions in Louisiana. Visiting him was one of the hardest things for me. The sound of metal on metal from handcuffs and foot shackles are sounds I will never forget. The mere sight of him cheesing from ear to ear as he walked up to me in his orange jail suit, despite being on lockdown 23 hours a day, was heartbreaking. His smiling exemplified my brother's optimistic character – another thing I will never forget.

He kept busy by writing us daily, narrating movies, and creating music. He started writing a book about his experiences and wanted to name it *Life Lessons*. And, since he didn't have a chance to finish high school before he was arrested, he earned his GED while in prison as well.

I still remember the first time I went to visit him in prison. He wanted to sing a new song that he had written. He made a clicking sound by beating on the prison countertop, and started singing a song he called "Love."

Tears flowed from my eyes. I never knew my brother could sing. I could tell, however, that he had been practicing for a while and was pretty excited about it. I was excited for him too – he clearly had an incredible talent.

He went on to write over 50 songs while incarcerated, and eventually hooked up with several top local artists in the area once he was released. He even performed in front of hundreds of people at a local concert, singing his hit song, "Love." The same song he had once sung to me while in prison became a local hit. It received back-to-back spins on the Shreveport radio station.

Halfway through his five-year sentence, Jonathan was allowed to participate in a program where he could work, but would still be considered a prisoner. Essentially, the program allowed him to work and live in a house with other inmates, who were also soon to be released. This was a way to prepare inmates financially and mentally for leaving prison, to begin the process of reintegrating back into society. Studies show that such programs reduce the risk of recidivism when compared to those released directly back into society, which, for some, could have been after ten years or more.

My brother's job had him working in a factory that chopped and sold wood. From the few conversations I had with Jonathan, I learned he was working long hours around a lot of wood dust, breathing it in without a mask. We never discovered whether that was what caused him to start getting sick. I just know that I received a call one day while at work saying that he wasn't doing well.

Jonathan was working at the factory when he suddenly became short of breath. When he went home to sleep at night, it became worse. He blew it off for a day or so, thinking it was just a common cold, but the shortness of breath wouldn't dissipate. Since he was technically still incarcerated, he was forced to hold out until his halfway house finally agreed to take him to the hospital.

What we found out, when he finally arrived at the hospital, was a shock to us all.

At the hospital, they took several x-rays and a CAT scan. These showed that he had fluid around his lungs and heart. It turned out his lung had collapsed from all the fluid compressing it. He was basically walking around with one functional lung. In order to remove the fluid from his lung, the doctors inserted a chest tube – a long, plastic, cylindrical device that is designed to drain fluid and re-inflate the lungs. Three liters of excess fluid, that had been compressing his lung, was drained. He was then taken into surgery for an emergent pericardiocentesis – a procedure where a tube is placed in the sac surrounding the heart, to remove excess fluid. After that, Jonathan was transferred to the intensive care unit for close monitoring.

In one of the many letters he wrote to me, he described this time as, "One of the most frightening times of my life. I have a tube in my nose, IV's in both of my arms, a monitor on my finger, a tube in my lung, one in my chest, and a drainage device for my urine. At one point, I thought I was going to die and I kept wondering why is all of this suddenly happening to me."

Since he was still considered a prisoner, an armed officer was required to sit by his side during his entire hospitalization. His hands and feet were chained to the hospital bed. During his ten-day stay in the ICU, we were not allowed to contact him. We could only call the nurse on duty, but they only gave us as little information as possible.

During his stay in the hospital, many tests were run. When they finally came back, we were shocked.

Jonathan was diagnosed with leukemia.

How could this have happened?

No one else in our family had cancer. Was it from the factory he had been working in for those past few years, breathing in all the dust without wearing a mask? Was the wood he worked around treated with chemicals that we did not know about?

We never truly learned what caused it, but when the cancer hit him, it hit him hard.

The chemotherapy drugs hit him even harder.

Losing his hair and weight and dealing with constant diarrhea were all signs the chemotherapy drugs were killing off the bad cancer cells. Unfortunately, it also meant his good cells were being killed in the process. Still, during that time, I never once heard my brother complain about his condition. He basically kept saying that he would beat it and become a millionaire.

LSU Hospital in New Orleans specialized in his condition, so he was transferred there for further care in 2008. New Orleans is five hours from my parents' place in Shreveport, Louisiana, which was the only problem. I was living in San Antonio, Texas at the time, serving in the military, and wasn't able to stay with him the whole time he received treatment.

One day, in early December 2008, something told me to go visit my brother in the hospital. At a moment's notice, I was on a plane heading to New Orleans. What I saw when I arrived forever changed the way I would treat and interact with patients on a day-to-day basis.

As I walked into Jonathan's room, all I could see were numerous IV lines and catheters. They seemed like they were coming from every orifice on his frail body. The thing about cancer cells is, as they are killed off with the chemotherapy, sometimes they can clog up your organs such as your kidneys and cause them to stop working. It seemed like that was actually happening to my brother.

Jonathan moaned in pain and writhed constantly in his hospital bed. The cancer drugs were working, but unfortunately causing him a lot of pain and shutting down his kidneys. I begged the nurse to give him something for the pain, but she explained with a shake of her head that he had already received pain meds. All I could do was just sit and watch my little brother lay helpless in pain. But he kept saying, "I will beat this, I will beat this."

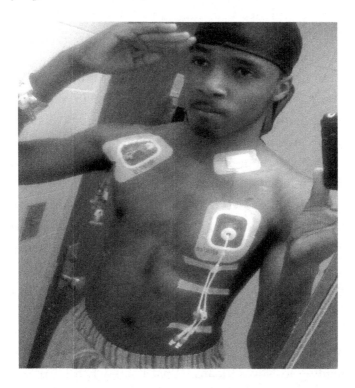

Despite being sick and receiving chemo, he always had a great sense of humor

I've worked in the hospital, while in the military, and have seen hundreds of patients lay sick in hospital beds. But, until that moment, I'd never had to see my own family sick and helpless like that. Seeing my brother in his hospital bed changed the way I approached and treated every patient from that point on. It changed my attitude toward my career and it changed my life.

I wasn't able to spend much time at the hospital during that trip. I had to leave a few days later, only to receive a phone call to inform me he wasn't doing well.

On December 8th, 2008, I was working in the Surgical ICU at Wilford Hall Medical Center in San Antonio, Texas when my phone rang. It was my aunt.

"Antonio, I'm so sorry but Jonathan has passed away."

My heart dropped to the ground, followed by my legs. I was vaguely aware of my coworkers looking around to see what was going on as I burst into tears – but I just couldn't hold it in. My best friend, my brother, my mentee, was gone. Just like that. Gone too soon.

At first I blamed myself. I wished I could have done more to keep my brother focused and headed down the right path in life. Perhaps, if I had spent more time with him, he wouldn't have hung around those guys and then wouldn't have ended up behind prison bars.

I will never get those five years he spent in prison back. I will never get my little brother back. All I know is that he is no longer in pain. Instead, he's looking down over me and smiling, just like he always was when I visited him behind those prison walls.

May you rest in peace, Jonathan Immanuel Webb
Sunrise: 28 June 1986
Sunset: 8 December 2008

"They can take away my freedom, but they can never take away my dreams." –Jonathan Immanuel Webb

ADVICE:

Be wary of who you call "your friend" and who you associate with. If you associate with people who are doing ungodly or illegal things, you might soon find yourself doing the same. All it takes is one mark on your record and your life will be scrutinized forever. Here are five signs that you may be hanging around the wrong crowd:

1. *When your friends are not supportive and try to discourage your dreams and goals*: Never let someone's opinion discourage your dreams. When I was applying to medical school, I met with my dean and several other school administrators, who were responsible for writing my letter of recommendation. I could hear discouragement in their voices when they told me they were unsure as to whether I would get accepted into medical school, let alone finish. Other people sometimes looked at me like I was crazy, when I told them I was applying to medical school and wanted to be a doctor.

Hang around people who will encourage and uplift you. Hang around people who see potential in you, even when you don't see it in yourself. Some people are very negative and never think outside the box. When they learn of your intentions, they try to persuade you and discourage you from reaching your goals.

The number three rule in the book, *48 Laws of Power* says to "conceal your intentions." Keep people off balance and in the dark by never revealing the purpose behind your actions. If they have no idea what you are up to, they can't prepare a defense. Lead them down the wrong path and by the time they figure out your true intentions, it will be too late.

2. *When your friends are around when times are good, but nowhere to be found when times get bad*: Will Smith said it best

when he said, "If you are absent during my struggle, don't expect to be present during my success." Over the years, I've come to realize who my true friends are. My true friends are those who I can go months without talking to, but still pick up right where we left off when we speak again. My true friends are there through the thick and thin.

When I was in medical school, there were times when I couldn't pick up the phone and call my friends or family for weeks at a time. During my second year of medical school, I once studied for 18-20 hours a day, for three days straight. I locked myself in my small apartment room and only came out for food and water. When I finally came out of hibernation, I had grown a beard and squinted the moment I stepped outside into the bright sun. I called my best friend and we picked up on a conversation where we left off a few days prior. Even when you don't speak for weeks or months at a time, true friends are always with you in spirit.

3. *When your friends observe you do something that may jeopardize your career and/or life and do not speak up:* Hang around people who will roughen you up and keep you straight, when you decide to venture off the right path. Those hardheaded guys, who robbed people as they were leaving ATMs with my little brother, were not his true friends. A true friend will not allow you to do something that would jeopardize your future or life. A true friend will give you a whack across your head after even a mention of something detrimental to your life or career. These individuals are your true friends. Find these individuals and keep them close.

4. *When your friends create and thrive off negativity:* Let's be honest, no one wants to be around someone who is always negative. The 'Debbie downer' of the group. The never satisfied friend or the friend that whatever you seem to do, it's not good enough. This person always finds something negative to say about every situation.

Hang around people who are positive and uplifting. The days when you are down, they lift you up and encourage you to never give up. There is a saying that goes, "You are the sum total of the five people you hang around with the most." So, which type of people are you most known to be around? Makes you think, doesn't it?

5. *When your friends' ideations and goals don't align with yours:* When my best friend wanted to go straight to college after high school and suggested I do the same, he could have gotten upset and ended our friendship when I refused. Real friends come to agreements and meet in the middle. Even though he really wanted us to go to college together, he understood where I was coming from and supported my decision of joining the military. A true friend will take the time to listen to your side of the argument and then try to understand where you are coming from.

Today, we still have disagreements. Usually over which stocks to invest in, but we mutually respect and value each other's input.

YOUNG AND AMBITIOUS

My very first job was selling watermelons on the side of the road in Louisiana. I was 15 and my older brother and cousin were both 17. It all started when we were eating at one of our favorite places in Louisiana, CiCi's Pizza, mainly because it was only $3 to stuff our faces with endless amounts of pizza. We made it our daily place to eat during the summer months.

One day while eating, we saw an older white gentleman getting out of an old, blue pickup truck. He had what seemed like hundreds of watermelons on the back of his truck. We all glanced at each other and thought to ourselves, *What's with all the watermelons?* I, in particular, became very curious and got up from eating to approach him.

"Are you *selling* those watermelons?" I asked him. He stood in line next to a younger white lady with dirty, blonde hair and short, cream-colored jeans. She looked at me and smiled, and then quickly looked away.

"Yes, we actually just moved here. We'll be selling them right on Mansfield Road," he stated.

Without thinking, I quickly asked, "Well, do you need any help selling them?"

We were all very ambitious, always trying to think of ways to make money. We would go from door to door to ask our neighbors if they needed their grass cut and accepted donations as payment. We even asked our neighbors if we could wash their cars for a few bucks.

One summer, we thought of a brilliant idea to design a fake school fundraiser. We printed out newsletters and fundraiser sheets to solicit the money. Then, we went from door to door and told people that we were raising money for a school trip to Washington,

DC. Some people slammed the door in our faces, but others showed us sympathy and graciously gave us a few dollars.

"Yes, actually, we could use some help. Here is my number. Call me first thing in the morning and you all can get started," he responded.

Wow! We were all very excited after hearing that. *We actually may have a legitimate job*, we thought. My dad, however, was somewhat concerned and skeptical about us working out in the heat for some old white man. After begging him for a while, he eventually agreed to let us do it and, to our surprise, we enjoyed it.

We initially started at one location, helping customers as they drove up to the tent. Our job was to stack the watermelons neatly, arranging the oldest watermelons in front and newest ones in the back. It was always hot outside but Mr. Charles, our boss, rewarded us with free watermelon at the end of each day. We got up bright and early each summer day and walked the two miles to our new job location. After a few weeks, we gained enough trust for him to leave us alone to sell watermelons by ourselves.

The business was booming!

People were buying watermelons so fast that Mr. Charles wanted to expand and set up several more locations around the city. He left my cousin at the main tent on Mansfield Road, me in his blue truck on another road, and my brother about ten miles away. Early in the morning, he dropped us off. At the end of the day, he picked us up and collected the day's profits. At times, I became very hungry and thirsty sitting in his blue pickup truck all day. Sometimes, customers caught me sleeping in the truck, as they stopped by to buy some watermelon.

Before that point, Mr. Charles never kept an inventory of how many watermelons he dropped off at each location with us. I soon realized this and started giving deals to customers. Instead of selling two watermelons for $7.00, I sold three for $8.00 and kept the extra dollar. I often spent the extra money on junk food at the corner store across the street. It didn't take long for Mr. Charles to realize that the amount of money he collected from us did not equal the number of watermelons sold. He then started counting the watermelons he dropped off with us, and made calculations at the end of the day. As a result, we were paid less because we could not give out the deals anymore.

A few weeks later, we decided that we did not want to work for Mr. Charles anymore and quit. Being out in the heat and working for someone else taught us many lessons that summer. Most importantly, we learned right away that we didn't want to work for someone else our entire lives.

WHAT I LEARNED FROM MCDONALDS

The legal age to begin working in the state of Louisiana is 16. I was only 15 at the time and eager to work, but knew it was pretty much impossible to get a *real* job at my age. One day, while walking home from school, I came up with brilliant idea. I thought if I could change the number two in '1982' to a one and make my birth year 1981, I would legally be 16. Then I could possibly get a job. Filled with excited, I rushed home with this idea. I was excited about all the money I would make, all the new clothes I would have and most importantly all the chicks I would get. My parents didn't have much and I knew my father would never pay $200 for a pair of Jordan sneakers. I knew that if I got a job, I could buy my own pair. I rushed home and was excited about my new plan. But, I had two obstacles in my way: to convince my dad to give me my birth certificate and to convince McDonalds to hire me with an altered birth certificate. After much back and forth talking, my dad finally agreed to let me copy my birth certificate.

I took the bus to the nearest library and asked to use their copier. After copying it, I used white out to change the 1982 to 1981, and made another copy of it. When the paper came out of the printer, I had a smile from ear to ear on my face and felt like I was printing real money. *This new birth certificate could open up many doors for me*, I thought. *I could get several jobs and never would have to rely on or beg anyone for rides and money*. I left the printer office and ran straight to McDonalds, asking to speak to the manager.

"Are you all hiring?" I stuttered and quickly realized that my voice came out sounding nervous and raspy.

"Not at the moment, but you can fill out an application and we will get back to you."

I was heartbroken. My plan fell through. What would I do now? There wasn't another McDonalds within walking distance from my house. And, I didn't have transportation to get to and from the next closest McDonalds. I felt like giving up, but filled out the application and turned it in anyway. A few days later, I returned to check on the status of the application and was met by a young black manager. His name was James and he seemed hip and cool. He had a sweet red two-door car outside, with some gold rims on it and a banging sound system. *Maybe if I played it cool, he would take me seriously and end up hiring me,* I thought.

"Can you interview now?" he asked.

I responded without hesitation. "Yes!"

What if he asked about my age? I thought. I've never had a real job before, besides selling the watermelons, nor had I ever been on a job interview. I'm sure he could sense the nervousness as he asked me question after question. But, whatever my responses were, they must have impressed him. I was offered the job right on the spot.

At age 15, I began my first *real* job and worked at McDonalds for two years, escalating in the ranks to shift manager.

I thought I had made it big!

Going to work in a shirt and tie and making $7/hour seemed luxurious to me at that point. Luxurious enough to ride a bicycle, which I bought from a friend for $25, to and from work. My dad was always busy and I didn't want to rely on my brother to pick me up and drop me off, so I figured the quickest and cheapest way to get to work would be on bicycle. This would get old fast as my shift sometimes ended when McDonalds closed at 1:00 am. Many times, I ended up riding home alone on the Louisiana dark streets. I knew the terrain and had a set route that I would take, but I also knew that I was in Louisiana and that anything could happen that late at night. Many times my bike broke down half way home and I would be stuck walking the rest of the way. Whenever this happened, I walked quickly and glanced over my shoulder every few minutes, to ensure no one was following me. Even to this day, I remember the frustration and tears as I rode home after those long nights of work, sweating from head to toe and reeking of hot grease and burger patties.

My family enjoyed the time that I worked at McDonalds though. Often, I would bring home food that was to be thrown away. Eating greasy burgers and fries late at night became our norm. Many times my father would put in special orders for food before I went to work, with me scrambling at the end of each night trying to fill those orders. I had no idea that years later, I would be taking and giving a different type of orders – orders given as a military non-commissioned officer in the United States Air Force.

ADVICE:

Just from looking at me, you would probably never have guessed that I once worked at McDonalds. Although it was a very stressful job for me and at many times I wanted to quit due to obnoxious customers and being under compensated, I learned many valuable lessons while working for McDonalds. Whether I was flipping burgers on the grill, sweeping and mopping the floors or working the drive through, I learned something from each task assigned. Friday nights, after high school football games, were often the busy nights. During these times, when many customers came in all at once, we relied on each other for support. Without teamwork, orders would not have been made, customers would have been upset, and we most likely would not have kept our jobs. This experience became vital years later during my time in the military when teamwork was essential to complete military missions. When I was promoted to shift manager, I supervised several employees, some of whom were twice my age. This gave me the opportunity to experience leadership at a young age.

In addition to leadership skills and learning the importance of teamwork, working for McDonalds taught me the value of saving and of the dollar. When I received my first paycheck from McDonalds, it was $93.07; although I felt like I had earned $900+ from all the hours I had worked. Before payday even arrived, I had several things planned out that I needed to pay for and wanted to buy. This forced me to learn how to effectively budget and save, starting from that first small paycheck. After some time, I saved up enough money to buy my first car — a 1984 Buick Riviera. I paid $600 for it from a used car dealership around the corner from my house. I was happy to get any car at all and thought I had gotten a good deal, even though the car had a big dent on the front bumper. The car had two doors and was as long as a school bus. It was beige brown in color, with chipped paint on the outside. The inside contained bucket seats that were ripped, along with a roof that was caving in. The lining of the seats looked like someone ran a knife through them, but I bought seat covers and never saw the rips again. I wanted to be like everyone else, so I had my friends' dad put in a stereo system with two loud 12" subwoofers that I purchased from a pawnshop. I didn't have money to spend on expensive rims, so I bought chrome hubcaps from a nearby tire shop. Even though they were not real rims, I kept them clean and polished so that they would shine. Having shiny wheels was a big deal back then. I thought that I was cool because after school, when everyone was outside waiting on their parents to pick them up, I turned up my bass loud and rolled in front of the school to "floss." Thankfully, the big dent that was on my front bumper was on the driver's side and everyone standing outside in front of the school only saw the passenger bumper. It was a good feeling to be able to save that much money and buy something on my own though. I was also glad that I didn't have to ride that darn bike to and from work anymore.

Whatever job you may be currently working, just know that it may only be a stepping-stone to your ultimate career and dream job. Several famous celebrities once worked at McDonalds. Fred Durst of Limp Bizkit, Amazon founder Jeff Bezos, and Jay Leno all once worked at McDonalds. Look around at your current job and ask yourself, what can I take from this job that will be valuable to me in the future? Next, learn as much as you can. Years later, you will look back and say, *Wow! I have come a long way.*

FAMILY IN PRISON

At one point, three of the six members of my family were in prison at the same time, all for different reasons. My brother was in prison on a juvenile life sentence for armed robbery. My little sister was in prison doing three years for two felony charges, and my mom was in prison for God knows what. As far back as I could remember from my childhood, my mom had been in and out of prison for various petty crimes that ranged from panhandling to trespassing. She was constantly on and off drugs. Every phone call I received from home was a nervous one. I was always prepared to hear the worse.

"Mom is in jail again," or "Mom has been missing for three days."

Whenever I heard this, I pretty much knew that she had either been arrested again, was out gambling, or was caught using drugs – crack cocaine – her drug of choice. To feed these habits, she often sold items from around the house or pawned gifts given to her by family members on holidays or birthdays. This made it difficult to send money for Mother's Day or give gifts on her birthday. I never knew whether I would be feeding into her vicious drug cycle or supporting her expensive gambling habit.

While growing up, my mom lived with her six other sisters in a small cozy house in a neighborhood of Shreveport called Queensborough. Her mother, my grandmother, struggled to raise them with the help of welfare and food stamps. And struggle they did. But, although they were poor, they didn't realize it because they were rich in happiness.

To earn money, my grandmother worked as a housekeeper for a rich white family in an affluent neighborhood of Shreveport called Highland Hills. She eventually started her own daycare business by adding two additional rooms onto the back of her house. She then used these rooms for her daycare business. She negotiated with the person who built the rooms and agreed to watch his grandson, in return for the weekly payments she would have made to him. In addition to watching other neighborhood kids, my grandmother watched my siblings and me. We usually went over to her house, while my dad was at work, so she could babysit us.

My mom attended Fair Park High School, a school not too far from her home in Queensborough. She did well in school, but her education was constantly interrupted by frequent visits to the hospital. Whenever an ambulance was called to the school, it was usually because of her. She always seemed to get sick, but no one knew why. Her sisters just knew that she was always in the hospital and on a lot of medications. They became curious.

"Why don't you take your medicine?" asked Lily, one of her older sisters who shared a bed with her.

"I do take it. I take it until I feel better and then stop. I just want to be normal."

Being normal was all that she wanted.

Imagine the kind of life circumstances that thrust you into adulthood, without having the time to mentally prepare for the responsibilities of being a mother, a wife, and a role model. That is the story of my mom. Emotionally devastating events occurred in rapid succession during her childhood. She became pregnant with my older brother at 17 years old. She was just a teen and young kid herself. Now, she had a child to care for. This was followed by marriage and the birth of three additional children. All of this may have overwhelmed my dear mother resulting in depression and a downward spiral of continual hospital stays.

Over the course of my childhood, I cannot recall thirty consecutive days when my mother was at home with my siblings and me. The overwhelmingly majority of the time she wanted to be there for us, but simply couldn't due to her frequent and repetitive visits to the hospital. I always knew that something was wrong with her, but I could never figure out what. And it wouldn't be until years later that I did.

Then, there was my dad.

The majority of my friends had fathers who were absent while they were growing up, either because they were in prison or were dead. My dad was just the opposite. He was a positive role model and was actively involved in our lives, but not before going through a troubled childhood himself.

FROM PRISONER TO MINISTER

My father was raised in a small poverty and drug stricken neighborhood in San Diego, called Logan Heights. From an early age, he experimented with hard drugs to get high. He used everything from LSD to Speed, and even sniffed glue to get high.

Though he grew up an only child, he was very close to his cousin, Chuck, who was like a brother to him. Chuck was a couple of years younger than my dad, and a big time drug dealer and gang member in San Diego. He lived in the southeastern part of the city, in a neighborhood called Skyline. Chuck constantly ran the streets and eventually found himself in turf wars with rival gang members.

One evening, Chuck was awakened by banging on his front door and a loud commotion outside. He looked out the front window and saw three guys standing on the porch, pacing back and forth.

"Chuck, come outside. We need to chat."

Chuck was skeptical and knew something was up, but grabbed his gun and headed outside anyway. The men led him towards a blue minivan that was parked on the curb. Just as they approached, the door of the van opened up.

"Shoot him!" screamed one of the gang members standing outside the van. "Shoot him!"

Chuck reached for his gun but before he could pull it out, two shots tore through his chest and he collapsed on the ground.

The shooter quickly moved to stand over him and pointed the shotgun at Chuck's face. Still gasping in pain, Chuck jerked his left arm over his face as more rounds from the shotgun were fired. His arm was instantly shattered into pieces.

But he *lived.*

Chuck underwent several surgeries and eventually received a prosthetic arm. The fake metal arm always frightened my siblings and me when he visited us in Louisiana. I often caught myself staring at it when he spoke, as if I was unable to tear my thoughts away from the horrifying story behind the limb.

The saddest part of Chuck's story was that he returned to the drug game after he recovered from his brush with death.

Weeks later, he was found *dead* in his home.

But, Chuck's death wouldn't slow down my dad. He continued to use drugs and commit crimes, which led to multiple run-ins with the law. In between breaking into people's houses and heavy drug use, my dad played football and ran track – and he was pretty good at it, too. In fact, he was so good that he was recruited to play football by The University of California, San Diego State University, Arizona State University, and by Coach Robinson at Grambling State University. He never made it to Louisiana, though, due to his troubled past. Instead, he put his speed and talent towards running from the cops as they chased him up and down the streets of San Diego.

"Stop right there you n!gger or I'll shoot!" shouted a middle aged, and distinctly white officer, with a belly that sunk far below his belt line. He drew his weapon quicker than a cowboy in a standoff.

My dad had just broken into a house that belonged to a white couple and stolen a radio, when – out of nowhere – a passing neighbor spotted him. They immediately called the police. My dad panicked at the thought of being caught and sent to jail, so he ran out the back door, dodging bullets aimed at his back and legs as the officer fired his 9mm weapon.

Lucky for my father, he escaped that time. But he didn't learn his lesson. He repeated the same process of breaking and entering over 20 more times, stealing anything he could get his hands on. During one particular break in a group of white guys, who were outside drinking, saw him climbing out a window and started to chase him.

The men yelled for the police, who happened to be nearby. The two officers also joined in on the chase. My dad ran across the street, with the stolen items in hand, and tried to find a quick escape route. He climbed on top of a roof, in a dark alley near University of California at Berkeley, and hid. His heart raced, while he prayed he wouldn't be spotted.

"You black ass s.o.b! You'll get 20 years! Put your hands where I can see them and come down."

Scared and out of breath, my dad finally gave in.

Once he was on the ground, he was thoroughly searched, handcuffed, and booked by the Oakland police department. At sentencing, several witnesses were present – each with their own account and description of my dad. Up until that point, he had always managed to get away with his crimes – but that time would be the last.

The judge tied him to several other crimes around the city and sentenced him to a year in jail. During his stint in prison, my dad passed time by drawing, writing, and talking with his mom, who came to visit every few weeks. Despite a few scuffles with other inmates and *constant* mouthing back to guards, he mostly stayed out of trouble and even obtained his GED while in prison.

After he served his time, he was invited to a place that would forever change his life: church revival.

Mr. Sam was the name of the man who invited my dad to church. He was an older gentleman and had been very ill, until a pastor prayed for him. It was then that he beat all the doctor's expectations and lived just long enough to reach out to my father.

During the revival, my dad gave his life to God and was forever changed, leaving his past of burglary, crime, and drug usage where it belonged – behind him.

Mr. Sam passed away soon after.

Everything you do happens for a reason. Everyone you meet comes into your life for a reason. And the effect people leave on others can ripple through lifetimes and generations. If that gentleman hadn't lived long enough to invite my dad to church, I most likely would not be writing this book today. My dad would have likely been killed while committing a crime or serving the remainder of his life in jail.

As soon as his life was back on track, my dad joined the California Army National Guard. He transferred to the United States Air Force in the early 80s, where he stayed until his 1996 retirement in Louisiana. That was where he raised my three siblings and me, after a long and emotional divorce from my mom.

I didn't understand much growing up and didn't realize the seriousness of my mom's medical condition (and wouldn't until 10+ years later) but, even then, I knew it was taking a toll on their marriage.

"Put your hands up and get on the ground!"

"Get on the ground!"

The shouts of several military officers bombarded my dad as he came home from work one evening. He was met by several military officers, who had their guns drawn and aimed at him. It was like a reenactment of one of his worst memories.

"Wait, wait! What's going on?" my dad screamed back.

An officer stepped forward and explained that they had been called because my mom had barricaded herself in the upstairs bathroom, and had threatened to hurt herself.

It wouldn't be the last time my mom would try to commit suicide. And each time, she edged closer to succeeding. She went back and forth from slashing her wrists to overdosing on pills. It seemed to happen more frequently over the years and resulted in multiple trips to the hospital to visit her. Eventually, it resulted in the divorce of my parents while I was still very young.

There are few fathers that would have done what my father did after the divorce, but I'm glad he made the decision to keep my siblings and me together. He didn't want to split us up or send us away to live with distant family members or in foster homes. He figured it would be best if we all stayed together, even though he knew it would be hard to raise four kids alone. He was more than ready to accept the challenge, if it meant keeping his family close.

Being in the military and on active duty entailed many responsibilities for my father. Luckily, the military understood. They allowed my father to take special duty assignments so we could be close to family members, such as my grandmother, who could watch us and help my father out. Financially, money was very tight. Living off a salary designed to support one to two people, my father did whatever he could to make it work and to make sure we had food on the table and clothes on our back.

One of the most powerful memories I have of my father is how he did whatever he could to make sure we had food to eat. More than once, he went around Louisiana and spoke at small churches, on street corners, or wherever he could preach the gospel and tell his testimony. He accepted small donations, which he used to support us.

Every few days for years, my dad donated his plasma for money. Getting $25-$30 for a one or two hour donation session sometimes seemed the only way to make ends meet. My siblings and I enjoyed going with my father, so we could eat the snacks that were given to the plasma donors in order to keep them from becoming hypoglycemic after donating. It was not until years later did I realize what my father was doing, and the extreme sacrifices he was making.

Another thing that always impressed me was my father's willingness and eagerness to help others who were less fortunate. Christianity was stressed in our household, and many things that we did growing up evolved around church. My dad eventually became the pastor of a small church in Marshall, Texas and ran the church for several years. On Saturdays, many members of our church ventured out into the community and handed out free food.

We also handed out Christian pamphlets and ministered to the people. I never understood why my father had such a strong desire to help others, when we were struggling ourselves. But, it instilled a mentality of altruism and a spirit of giving that I am grateful for, even to this day.

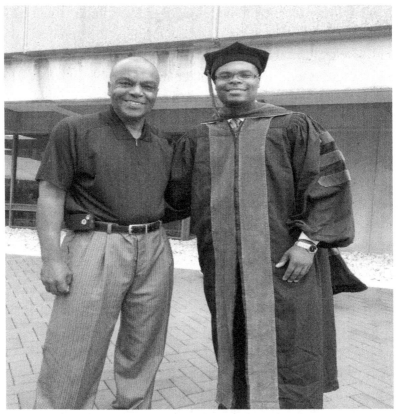

Me and Pops

ADVICE:

The greatest gift a father can give to a child is to be in his or her life! Studies show that fathers who are involved in their children's life bring positive benefits that no other person is likely to bring. The children with involved and caring fathers tend to have better educational outcomes, linguistic and cognitive capacities, and verbal skills. In addition, they tend to have higher IQs along with academic achievement that carries well into adolescence. A study in 2001, by the U.S. Department of Education, found that highly involved biological fathers had children who were 43 percent more likely than other children to earn mostly A's and 33 percent less likely than other children to repeat a grade. Conversely, when a father is absent, it negatively impacts the child in several ways. Studies show that an absent father lowers a child's educational attainment and decreases the likelihood that they will graduate from high school. Children with absent fathers are more likely to smoke cigarettes and use drugs or alcohol. In addition, they have five times the average suicide rate, increased rates of depression, increased incarceration rates, and lower average incomes.

I commend and applaud those of you out there who are stepping up to the plate and taking care of your children. And, if you are not, it's never too late to begin! Here are several tips on how to be a great dad:

- *Spend time with your children:* when you add up all the time your child spends in daycare, in school, asleep, at the babysitters or otherwise occupied with activities that don't include you, the remaining time becomes precious. There are 940 Saturdays between a child's

47

birth and the time he or she leaves for college. If your child is already five years old, about 260 of those Saturdays are already gone. Make each Saturday count. Take your children for a walk, play with them at the park, and attend their sporting events. They will remember this and cherish it forever.

- *Respect your children's mother:* One of the most important influences a father can have on his child is an indirect one. Fathers influence their children in large part through the quality of their relationship with the mother of their children. A father who has a good relationship with the mother of his children is more likely to be involved and more likely to spend quality time with his children. This means children who are psychologically and emotionally healthier. When children see their parents respecting each other, they are more likely to feel like they are also accepted and respected. If you are married, the best thing you can do is to be a good husband to your children's mother. It teaches them how to behave once they do get married, and prepares them for a successful marriage. If you are not living with or are not with your children's mother, your children may miss out on the opportunity to observe those little moments shared between a husband and wife that show respect and love. At the end of the day, she is still their mother and regardless of the differences between you two, you will want your children's future behavior to be modeled by yours.

- *Be a role model:* Your children look up to you, whether you realize it or not. When my dad was struggling day in and day out to make sure we had food on the table and clothes on our backs, I noticed how hard it was for him. I could tell when he was stressed out, when money was low, or when he was having a bad day. He didn't have to say a word – I noticed it through his actions. Children are always watching and are gifted observers. They rely more on nonverbal messages than on words. The wonderful thing about raising your children is that it allows you to share the best parts of your own childhood, and perhaps to give your children the things you never had. The values and morals that I possess, even to this day, came from my father's teaching and wisdom over the years. I will be forever grateful.

- *Read to your children:* reading to your children has several benefits. Children are always on the go – constantly running, playing, and exploring the environment. Snuggling up with a book allows for the two of you to build a stronger relationship. Numerous studies have shown that students who are exposed to reading before preschool are more likely to do well in all facets of formal education. Reading teaches basic speech skills, the basics on how to read a book, better communication and logical thinking skills. I vividly remember the summers when my parents made my siblings and I go to the library and read books. We went primarily because when we read a certain number of books, we received free Churches Chicken coupons. Nonetheless, it got us in the habit of reading and kept us off the streets of Louisiana when we were very young. As a parent, reading to your children is one of the most important things you can do to prepare them with a foundation for academic excellence.

DON'T QUIT NOW

Antonio, let me know what you plan to do. You have to make a decision now, but realize whatever decision you make will affect you for the rest of your life. You made it this far, don't quit now."

I looked over at my dad, who had come to a meeting with my high school principal and I, and saw tears coming down his face. Before that moment, I never once saw my father cry. They say it takes a lot for a grown man to cry. And, I was certainly putting my dad through a lot. I knew then how much my choices had affected my dad and how much he didn't want me to drop out of school.

The truth was, I had contemplated that very thing. The meeting between my father and the principal was to discuss my future plans. They arranged for all three of us to meet, after I verbalized my desire to drop out of school.

My main issue was with my school requiring me to attend class, when all my graduation requirements had been met. My school was on a quarter system, so mid-way through my senior year of high school, I completed all requirements for graduation. In my opinion, it seemed cruel to still make me go to class every day, especially since they were boring classes like Art. I didn't want to be in class and everyone knew it, including my Art teacher, Mr. Rogers.

Mr. Rogers was one of the school's few older, black teachers. He was known for his infamous jerry curl. The students, myself included, used to always joke and kid about how much gel he had in his hair. It always seemed to shine and glisten, like he drenched his head in activator juice before coming to class each day. He had me placed in ISS (In School Suspension) because apparently, he didn't appreciate me "acting out" in class and being disruptive. He also had talks with my father, who worked security at the same high school. Security was one of the few jobs he could get after retiring from the military, without a college degree. I knew better than to "act up" at school. All my teachers had to do was call my dad, and he would take care of me when we got home. But, that time I didn't care that he had me placed in ISS or that he had a long talk with my dad about me being disruptive in class. I had reached my breaking point. I just didn't care to be in school anymore.

My plan to drop out seemed ingenious at that point. I wanted to move to Houston, work several jobs, and make lots of money. Being in Louisiana, I was around a lot of drug dealers and people who got money from hitting licks. This meant I was constantly bombarded with the flashy lifestyle of nice cars, big rims, fancy clothes, Jordan shoes, and jewelry – everything a young kid from Louisiana could dream of. And, I wanted to be a part of it. I figured that once I dropped out of high school, I would move in with my aunt in Houston and save up money. Once I made it big, I'd come back to Shreveport and "floss" or show off to everyone.

At the time, it really did seem like the perfect plan. But, once I saw my father's tears, those images were immediately erased. I didn't need any more encouragement to stay focused for the rest of the year. I went to class each day, even though it seemed useless.

I still had one other problem – I needed to get out of Shreveport. The crime in the area started to pick up and before long, I was back hanging out with the wrong crowd again. I don't recall what I did to upset some gang members, but one day they came to my sister's job at the mall with guns looking for me. They asked where I was and told my sister they were going to kill me. As far as my other friends, it seemed like majority of them were getting killed or locked up. I knew that in order to avoid this from happening to me, I needed a way to get out of Shreveport. Otherwise, I would have become another statistic - just another black male dead or in prison.

ADVICE:

School and education are the most important investments you can make in yourself, so don't quit or give up! Dropping out of school is not cool, nor does it mean that you are grown up or more mature. In fact, it makes you the exact opposite. If you are contemplating dropping out, consider these facts:

1. High school dropouts have a life span that is nine years shorter than people who graduate.
2. According to the U.S. Census Bureau, dropouts are more likely to face poverty and a life filled with financial obstacles.
3. Dropouts are eight times more likely to go to prison than non-dropouts.
4. Nationally, 68 percent of state prison inmates are dropouts.
5. High school dropouts nearly universally come to *regret* their decision later in life.

You've probably have had enough of boring classes in school (like I did with my Art class), and you probably think that school has nothing to do with real life. You want to make real money and want it NOW! Usually, this leads down a path of making money the illegal way. Fast money is not always the best money. Being around drug dealers and people who hit licks to get money creates a false illusion of a lifestyle that appears to be glamorous and lavish. Who doesn't want this type of lifestyle? I know I sure did while growing up, and I started making irrational decisions because of it. I was blinded by what I saw the dope boys doing. They had the biggest rims on their cars, most expensive whips, nicest clothes, and all the girls. This is called "smoking and mirrors" and many people fall for this trap. They are drawn in by what they see, and don't realize the type of lifestyle that comes with it. Most of the drug dealers I grew up with always carried a gun and constantly looked over their shoulder everywhere they went. Every knock on the door sent them into frantic escape mode.

Years ago, I was hanging out at a friend's house in Shreveport when someone knocked on the door extremely hard. We were just hanging out and watching TV. Several pounds of weed were on the dining room table and three large guns were nearby. The guy, whom the drugs belonged to, freaked out when he heard the banging on the door and ran straight for his guns and weed. He quickly darted to the back room and hid them under his bed. Everyone else ran towards the back door to escape. I almost tripped over someone while running towards the door. Turns out, it was the neighbor coming by to drop off some mail. Months later, we thought it hilarious when we joked about it, but it was scary to think that the police could have been at the door that day and sent us all to jail. Do you really want to live your life like this? Instead, stay in school and earn money the legal way. It will last longer.

If I would have dropped out of high school, I would not be a doctor today. Individuals who drop out of high school have a harder time getting a good, secure, decent paying job. Most entry level and trade specific jobs require a minimum of a high school diploma. Studies show that non-degree holders can expect to earn 75% less than a bachelor's degree holder, who can expect to earn 2.7 million over their lifetime. A Master's degree will earn you 2.67 million while a doctoral degree can earn you 3.65 million over your lifetime.

According to a study by US Money News, some of the best jobs that pay $80k+ per year include: Art Director ($95,000/year), Business Operations Manager ($114,490), Civil Engineer ($82,710/year), Computer Systems Analyst ($82, 320/year) and Financial Analyst ($87,740).

A study by an international wealth consultancy group, called Wealthinsight, interviewed almost 70,000 millionaires worldwide to see what college degrees they held. At the top of the list was an engineering degree, which has resulted in more millionaires worldwide than any other degree.

Engineers are said to be innovators. They have the ability to create new and valuable products. If this is combined with an entrepreneurial spirit, engineers have the potential to become very successful. An example would be a Mechanical Engineer. These engineers design, build, and test mechanical devices like tools, machines, and engines. Mechanical Engineers have a median annual salary of $80,580, according to the Department of Labor. Not millionaire status, but certainly not bad.

Ranked in at number two was a Masters in Business Administration (MBA). The objective of business is to make money, so having an MBA would only make sense to achieve a number two on the list. A few of my classmates actually took a year off from medical school to get a dual MD/MBA degree. The degree is designed to help people lead companies and it usually pays off in the long run. An example would be a Financial Manager. These professionals plan and direct the financial arm of organizations to ensure they remain successful and healthy. And, while this occupation may not have you sitting upon millions of dollars yourself, you may still be able to make a substantial pile of green. Financial Managers have a median annual salary of $109,740.

The number three degree that produced the most millionaires was a Bachelors degree in Economics. Having this degree allows you to understand how to buy and sell. With this understanding, you can go into a wide variety of fields or start your own business. An example would be a Budget Analyst. These professionals help both public and private companies organize their finances by analyzing and strategizing budgets. While this role is all about the flow of money, don't assume you'll be getting your millionaire membership card just yet. Budget analysts have a median annual salary of $69,280.

Don't get me wrong, you don't have to have a degree to become successful. Everyone knows the story of Bill Gates, who left behind the books at Harvard University, but is now worth $66 billion. Or Facebook founder, Mark Zuckerberg; He dropped out of Harvard University in 2004, during his sophomore year, to work on Facebook full time. He is now worth over $16 billion dollars. Then there is Whole Foods owner, John Mackey, who dropped out of the University of Texas several times, never graduated, and never took a course in business. Twenty-five years later, Whole Foods has gone international and does more than $12 billion in sales.

I've met many people over the years that just go to school because their parents make them or because everyone else is doing it. These are wrong reasons to go. The decision to go to school has to come from within you. Ultimately, you have to make the decision. Think about what you want out of life, not what others want from you. You will be the one taking out loans, putting in all the hours, and getting up each morning to head to work. Make it your decision, not someone else's.

Take some time and do research on potential career fields. Instead of trolling on Facebook, take ten minutes and google the nearest hospital or fire station to your home and ask for shadowing opportunities. When I wanted a research position in medical school, I emailed ten different people at the same time. Basically the same email, just worded and addressed differently to each person. All it takes is one person to email you back. Don't get discouraged when the only person you emailed doesn't get back with you. Email them again or email him/her along with ten other people, as backups.

SECTION II:
Military

BOOT CAMP

One afternoon, after a long day of classes, my best friend suggested that we apply for scholarships and go to college together. After much thought, I politely refused.

"I'm going to join the military. It'll give me a way to pay for college and I'll gain medical experience in the process," I told him.

He looked confused, as if I had said I was going to jump off the Red River Bridge or something. I waited for a negative response, but it never came. Instead, he just nodded his head and accepted my plan. We then went on with our day.

My family has a strong history in the military. My father initially served in the US Army and later transferred to the US Air Force. His dad – my grandfather – served in the US Air Force, and my older brother joined the Army right out of high school. He has since graduated from college and is now a Captain in the US Army.

It was only right that I continued my family tradition of military service. On January 16, 2001, during the middle of my senior year of high school, I signed on the dotted line. Since I was 17 at the time, my father had to cosign for me to join. I was sworn in and vowed to defend my country. I left behind my comfort zone of friends and family in exchange for loud-yelling drill sergeants and immaculate, spit shined military boots. The infamous Reveille bugle 4:00 am wake up sound, 5:00 am three-mile runs, and M-16 weapons quickly became the norm for me.

The six weeks of boot camp flew by, and somehow I managed to stay out from under the radar of Sergeant Luston, my drill sergeant. Sergeant Luston was a tall white gentleman, no older than 26, who always rocked a high and tight military haircut. He had only been a drill sergeant for six months prior to taking on our flight. If I thought my dad's militaristic house rules were strict, I had another thing coming. Boot camp was intense and very structured. Firm military style rules were enforced. Our beds had to be made perfectly, with square hospital corners, and without wrinkles. Our socks and underwear had to be folded neatly and placed in our lockers. Our boots had to be shined and glistening, and our faces had to be teenage pre-puberty age shaven. A single dust mite located anywhere near our belongings resulted in several minutes of obscene and vulgar yelling while we stood at military attention. I often enjoyed it when the drill sergeants yelled and got into the faces of my fellow trainees and called them every single name in the book. The drill sergeants didn't like my smirking too much though, but I found it humorous. It helped me get through those six *long* weeks.

Each week presented a new challenge and obstacle to overcome. Our first week was called "zero week." It was spent in processing – getting military style, bald haircuts called "buzz cuts" and assigned to specific dorms. We were then divided to form specific flights, which consisted of 50-60 other trainees. During zero week, our flight was called the "Baby flight" or "Rainbow flight." This is because before we received our uniforms, everyone wore civilian clothes of various colors. When we congregated, the assorted colors resembled a rainbow. The following week, we received our military uniforms and got the dreaded shots in our butts. *Man!* Receiving those shots was incredibly painful – but not as painful as watching the trainees in front of you receive theirs as they squirmed in agony.

Every morning consisted of a 3:50 am wakeup call from the loudspeakers. Within ten minutes, we were expected to be up, dressed, and shaven. Our beds were expected to be perfectly made and ready for inspection by our drill sergeant. After a while, we came up with a brilliant idea. We thought it would be clever to sleep on top of our blankets. Then it would us save time in the morning, instead of rushing to make our beds and get everything done before inspection time. The plan didn't last long though, because our drill sergeant quickly caught on. In response, he flipped over my neighbor's bed. He then made him make it over, while he yelled at the poor guy for ten minutes straight.

At the halfway point of boot camp, we underwent the dreaded "Red Line Inspection." Essentially, this entailed a thorough inspection of every dorm by the head drill sergeant. Before the inspection, we conducted "dust drills," where we attempted to remove every speck of dust from every possible part of our dorm. This meant dusting our dorm from top to bottom, on our hands and knees. Any microscopic sight of dust resulted in ten minutes of excessively loud disciplinary screaming, while standing at parade rest.

Our wall lockers also had to be kept a specific way. Uniforms were required to be kept on the left side of the wall locker and our field jacket and physical training clothes on the right. Our clothing drawer contained our towels, each with our last name written in black marker. It also contained our underwear, brown military t-shirts, and socks. Each dorm received demerits from the inspection and these were tallied to calculate a total score. At the conclusion of boot camp, an honor flight was selected.

Each morning at 4:00 am, we met outside on the training pad for PT (physical training). We then ran three to four miles followed by pushups, sit-ups, jumping jacks, and flutter kicks. We appreciated the early run time because by 8:00 am, the Texas heat became unbearable and was a recipe for heat strokes and dehydration.

At 5:00 am, we headed to the cafeteria, which we called the "Chow Hall." Even though we always looked forward to eating, it was like walking on thin ice the whole time. Our every movement was scrutinized and made a mockery of by a slew of drill sergeants in the pit. The pit was where the drill sergeants hung out and ate. It was strategically placed directly in front of chow hall, so that our every move could be seen. Any incorrect foot positioning, while marching, or any violations of the dress code meant several minutes of excessive yelling followed by embarrassing looks from fellow trainees. I found it best to avoid eye contact with the drill sergeants in the pit and instead concentrated on looking serious, straight ahead, and focused.

At 5:20 am, we headed to lecture. We learned about military history, Air Force planes, and military customs and courtesies. We also were taught the Air Force's three core values: Integrity first, Service before self, and Excellence in all that we do. These core values served as the standard for our behavior and were meant to guide us through our military careers.

In the evenings, after class, we practiced marching in formation. This was done in order to perfect marching together as a flight, in preparation for graduation day and inspection. Sharp, crisp commands from our drill sergeant and snapping sounds from our combat boots hitting the drill pad, could be heard echoing across the parade grounds. The marching drills and countless hours of practice, in 100-degree heat, were designed to provide us with more than just the frustration from constantly being yelled at. They were designed for us to develop an instinct for precision and an ingrained habit of obedience to command. In addition, they aimed to instill habits that would provide the foundation of discipline, alertness, and quick response – traits essential in peacetime and during war.

At exactly 9:00 pm each night, military taps was played over the loudspeakers. This was followed by lights out. We then repeated the exhausting process. Every day. For six weeks.

Our final week of boot camp was called Warrior week, which consisted of a week spent out in the field. We completed a two-mile confidence course, stayed in tents to mock a real deployment, shot M-16 rifles, played war games with camouflage face paintings, and received field tactic instruction by security forces. We essentially learned the basic survival skills that would be needed in a wartime situation. The confidence course consisted of twenty obstacles designed to test strength, endurance, and willpower. It was also the time when we developed team-building skills. We often cheered each other on for encouragement throughout the long course.

At the rifle range, we were required to fire at man-sized targets from 75, 180 and 300 yards while lying, standing, and kneeling. I quickly found out that I needed to shoot with my left hand, even though I am right handed. That was because I couldn't close my left eye by itself, while leaving my right eye open, in order to look down the barrel of the rifle. That was probably the reason I didn't qualify as an expert shooter or receive an extra medal, called the 'Small Arms Expert' ribbon. The medal was given to trainees who displayed accuracy and precision while firing at the targets.

We also learned the basics of surviving in harsh conditions, particularly in combat. We were then evaluated on this training with mock exercises, called "war games." Our war games were taken very seriously. Being off guard, even for one second, meant being taken out by a sniper or stepping on a live grenade. But, unlike in actual war, the snipers were our drill sergeants with fake M-16 weapons and the grenades were plastic devices placed strategically around our camp. Our drill sergeants, however, attempted to make everything else about the war game as realistic as possible. There were loud speakers, which played sounds of gunshots being fired and explosions from grenades. There were also four-foot high bunkers made out of sandbags, assigned guards to protect our fort, a guard tower, and a stockade. During the middle of our war game, we were challenged with the task of donning our MOPP (Mission Oriented Protective Posture) gear and going into the gas chamber. The MOPP gear consisted of a gas mask, multiple thick layers of garments, M9 detector paper which detects chemical agents, gloves and boots. Having that gear on in the hot Texas heat meant there was a chance of dehydrating very quickly. Before even going into the gas chamber, some people passed out from heat exhaustion. Once in the gas chamber, we took off our gas masks and were required to state our full name and social security number. We often got stuck in the middle of our phrases, because the gas was so strong. The key was to not breathe in through your mouth. But, having to yell your name and social security number to the drill sergeant made this nearly impossible. Afterwards, we ran out of the chamber as quickly as possible, burning in agony and immediately vomiting and spitting up. The gas burns any open areas on the body including the chest, neck, ears and eyes. It also makes your nose run profusely, like a broken faucet.

The conclusion of the week meant two things: a five-mile road march, with a 60-pound rucksack on our backs, and receiving our Airman's coin. Receiving this coin embarked the journey of being called an Airman. It also meant the successful completion of basic military training.

I successfully completed boot camp on March 5, 2001 and returned to Shreveport just in time for my high school graduation. My friends and family were excited to see me return in one piece. I lost about eight pounds from all the running and limited amounts of food, but I was happy to be back and thrilled about finishing high school.

I finished high school in the top 5% of my class and with Honors. I was also able to walk the stage, to receive my diploma, in full military uniform with the rest of my classmates. In addition, I successfully completed the Fair Park Medical Careers Magnet program, a prestigious program at a nearby local high school that chose students based off academics and recommendations. The program introduced high school students to the career opportunities in medicine and other healthcare fields. Those in the program took extra science and anatomy courses, visited local medical schools, attended health symposiums, and participated in mock mass casualty exercises, where I often played the sick patient.

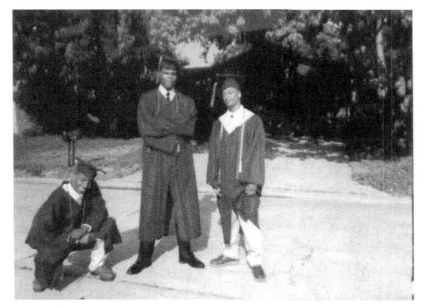

Me, in my military dress uniform before graduation, and my two best friends

This program essentially changed my trajectory in life and ultimately sparked my interest in going into medicine. At that point, I knew I wanted to be a doctor and vowed to do everything possible to make it happen. But, I had one obstacle in my way: military orders to Iraq.

ADVICE:

Joining the military was one of the best decisions I made in my life. Ultimately, it got me off of the rough streets of Louisiana and allowed me to gain medical experience while obtaining a way to pay for college. During my eight years in the military, the military paid for three Associates degrees and a Bachelor's degree. They also paid for my books, fees, and supplies. Once I left the military, I was still entitled to tuition assistance, which I used to fund part of my medical school. I received a stipend of $1906 every month, just for serving and completing my commitment with the military. I used this for housing expenses and food. At the age of 21, I purchased my first house with the help of the military. I utilized a VA loan, which required no money down. I also received a fixed, low 30-year interest rate. I currently still own that house in Texas and rent it out to other military members. In addition, I was entitled to free medical and dental care through Tricare, the military's healthcare network. Whether I needed my tonsils taken out or my wisdom teeth pulled, the military took care of it with little or no cost on my end. After joining the military, one can expect some of the best healthcare, utilizing the newest technology, and numerous benefits that very few civilian employers can match.

You may be wondering which branch of the military would be best for you. There are five branches of the military, so deciding on a particular branch can become difficult. Each branch, however, plays a unique role in the security of our country.

The Air Force is the most recently established branch of the military, after becoming a separate branch in 1947. Its main purpose is to support the security of the United States through air and space exploitation. On the other hand, the Army is the oldest branch of the military. It was established in 1775 and is considered to be the ground force of the military. The Navy was also established in 1775 and is considered the defender of the seas. In terms of size, the Marines are the second smallest branch of the military, only bigger than the Coast Guard. The Coast Guard was established in 1790 and its primary focus is to control illegal immigration by sea and conduct sea rescues.

I may be partial, but the Air Force has been known to treat their troops the best and have the best base locations around the world.

Although there are a lot of perks and benefits of being in the military, if you are thinking of joining you must weigh and consider the cons. Whether you join the Air Force, Army, Navy, Marines, or Coast Guard you can expect to spend a significant amount of time away from your family and home. The average person in the Navy can spend a significant amount of time each year at sea. According to 2003 statistics, on any given day, 40 percent of Navy personnel are assigned to a ship or submarine, and 35 to 45 percent of those ships will be deployed to sea.

In the Air Force, depending on your job, you may find yourself spending up to four to six months every year deployed to areas such as Kosovo, Saudi Arabia, Kuwait, Afghanistan, or Iraq. I have friends in the Air Force that have been deployed to Afghanistan and/or to Iraq three to four times since we first joined. Even if you elect to join the National Guard or Reserves, these branches now spend a significant amount of time deployed to areas such as Iraq and Afghanistan.

While growing up, my dad spent a significant amount of time away from home. My siblings and I stayed with family members, usually my grandmother, while he was away. And, even though my dad couldn't be there to discipline us, my grandmother would. The times when we "acted up" or didn't listen to my grandmother, she made us go outside to pick out our own switch from a tree in her backyard. Once back inside, we received whippings with those very switches. It took us a while to catch on to the fact that the smaller switches actually hurt more than the larger ones. By the time we figured this out, we had already learned to behave while over at her house.

While in the military, my dad received orders for an unaccompanied tour to South Korea, where he lived for more than a year. He was then given orders to Anchorage, Alaska for a three-year assignment. The tour was unaccompanied – meaning his family wasn't allowed to go with him, even though it meant he would be away for a very long time. He often sent videos and gifts from Alaska and visited from Korea whenever he could. It was hard enough not having a mom in the house, but when my father kept getting sent away, it became even harder.

Consider the above when deciding whether to join the military. And know that when you sign on the dotted line, there's always a good chance you may be sent on an unaccompanied tour overseas or to war.

KABOOM

KABOOM! Missiles and rocket-propelled grenades flew in every direction over our makeshift hospital tent.

"Incoming!" The startling call was shouted over the loudspeakers as it was also announced that four wounded soldiers, with head trauma and shrapnel injuries, were en route to our field hospital. We rushed frantically to grab our weapons and to don our bulletproof vest and helmet.

We had been attacked, once again, by the Iraqi insurgents.

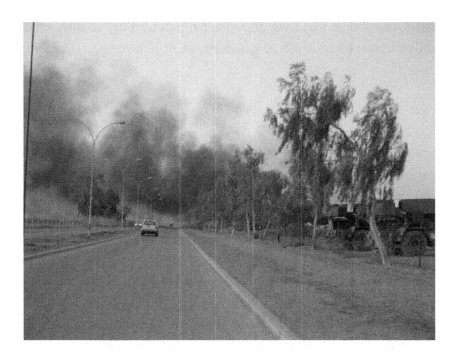

At that moment, I was in the Sunni Triangle 20 minutes from Baghdad, providing medical care in a 40-pound bulletproof vest and working in scorching 140-degree weather. Thoughts raced through my head. *How did I end up here? Will I make it out alive?*

Although such events seemed to occur daily, with no rest in between, we still worked diligently to do our job, dangerous or not. We were sent to Iraq to accomplish an important mission: to provide medical support for our American troops, Iraqi military personnel, and even Iraqi insurgents. But, in order to do that, we had to stay alive ourselves.

Fortunately, I managed to do just that. I spent an entire five-month tour in Iraq and lived to tell about it. Sadly, not every soldier in my rotation was as fortunate. I can say, however, that I did my part to save as many lives as I could. Receiving enemy gunfire and being shot at by RPGs (rocket propelled grenades) made a very difficult environment to do my job, but I didn't have a choice. I made a promise to myself, to the military, and to the American people that I would protect and defend my country when called upon. I had a job to get done, even if it meant risking my own life in the process.

....

Before leaving the US, my unit received multiple briefings from different experts about our upcoming deployment. My parents were worried for me, but they understood that I was the one who had ultimately signed on that dotted line. Military intelligence gave us a confidential briefing on where we would be going, what kind of combat we would be facing, and information on cyber security. We were instructed to not send or give away our location and to not make a daily broadcast of what we were doing over social media networks. During early 2005, MySpace was the popular social network and was a means to communicate easily with our families, updating them conspicuously about our well-beings. The last thing we needed was for the enemy to find out our arrival time into the country. That would have been a disaster waiting to happen.

We also received a briefing by Infection Control about the potential diseases we would be at risk for in the country. We received vaccinations and prophylactic medications against deadly diseases such as Yellow Fever, Typhoid, and Anthrax.

Briefing after briefing occurred as our anxious tensions rose. I was very young at that time – 20 years old – but had risen the ranks swiftly to become a Staff Sergeant non-commissioned officer. This meant I was an enlisted personnel but not commissioned. Most individuals who were officers and commissioned had bachelors or graduate degrees, allowing them to receive higher pay, with added responsibility in return. As a staff sergeant, I was responsible for directly supervising several younger airmen, ensuring their well-being was sought after, and to make sure they made it home from our deployment unharmed.

The whole event became surreal as we met with our families at the staging facility on base to say our last minute goodbyes. Wives were present, young children were running around oblivious to the fact that they may not see their mom or dad for months on end, and mothers and fathers were nervously giving last minute hugs and kisses. But it all came to a quick end when our families were forced to say one last goodbye. We then gathered in the auditorium for one final briefing.

After what seemed like hours, we concluded the briefing and boarded a military ambulance bus that was waiting for us outside. One by one we climbed aboard, with our gear in hand. I made my way to the back of the bus and met up with one of the medics from the hospital. He looked familiar. I was pretty sure I had seen him around the hospital a few times before, so I decided to sit next to him.

"You ready for this?" he asked.

"Yeah man, I'm just ready to get there and get to work," I said.

Before we could even finish the conversation, the bus departed and we began the drive to Kelly Air Force base, where our plane was waiting for our arrival.

Kelly Air Force Base is the oldest continuously operating flying base in the United States. The base has ties dated back to World War I, when it served as a training center for aviators, mechanics, and support personnel. The majority of the combat aviators of World War I earned their flying wings at Kelly Air Force Base. During the Iraq war, the military continued to use it as a docking location for troops heading into war.

We departed Kelly Air Force Base and began our 14-hour flight to the military's largest base in the Middle East, Al Udeid Air Base in Qatar.

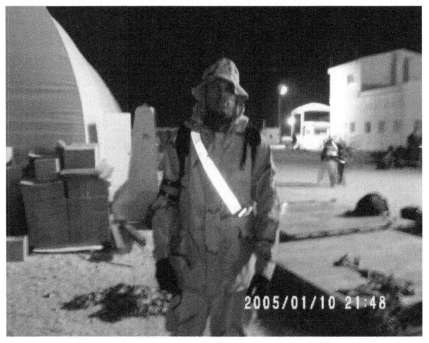

Qatar

Qatar is a sovereign Arab country located in Western Asia. It is bordered by Saudi Arabia to its south and surrounded by the Persian Gulf Sea. Most of the country consists of desolate miles of land, covered with sand. The average temperature in summer months can reach as high as 115 degrees. Despite these harsh conditions, Qatar is astoundingly rich. It is ranked as the world's richest country per capita and has the world's third largest natural gas and oil reserves in excess of 25 billion barrels.

Prior to heading into Iraq, Al Udeid served as our basing hub and staging facility. Historically, it was once considered a combat zone. An executive order from the president designated it as an area in which US armed forces engage or have engaged in combat in the past. For years, it had been safe and free of terrorism attacks. We were thrilled that even flying into the country for one minute meant that we would get the whole month of our pay tax free, since it was technically still considered a combat zone.

As we entered the country of Qatar, it didn't appear to resemble a combat zone. There was no fighting going on, no gunshots heard, and no rockets being fired. Just miles and miles of barren desert.

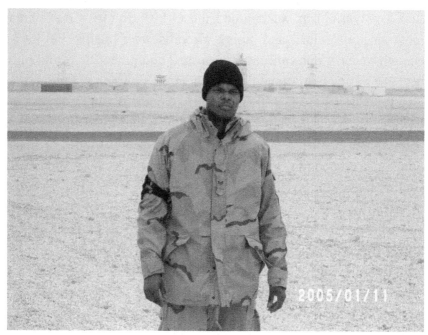

Al Udeid, Qatar

Hot, windy air blew into our faces the moment we stepped off the C-130 aircraft, as miles of the sandy desert surrounded us in every direction. We were only scheduled to be there for a few days, tying up some requirements and undergoing last minute training exercises before heading into war. We also spent a good amount of time eating at the cafeteria and hanging out in the recreation center, anxiously awaiting the word to depart.

In the military, there is the motto of "hurry up and wait" and the wait that day seemed like forever. It was a scorching 120 degrees that day in Qatar and a look around the room revealed that everyone was just as nervous as I was. I had never been to combat, and neither had most of the troops that were with me. Our plan was to wait until it became dark, so we could enter into the country while the insurgents were asleep.

The time to leave came at 2105. It was time to head into war.

I grabbed my gear, threw my weapon over my shoulder and said a prayer. Then we boarded the C-130 aircraft – one of the most uncomfortable and noisy aircrafts ever made, but large enough to carry our entire unit, gear and equipment. It would only be a one to two hour plane ride. *What could go wrong?* I thought.

The ride on the C-130 started off smooth. We initially just sat back and nervously looked at each other, because the loud engine of the plane drowned our voices when we tried to talk. To make things more uncomfortable, the back of the plane did not have air conditioning so it became very hot. It became so hot that I started to sweat through my uniform. So, I took off my bulletproof vest and set it on the ground near my boots.

It was dark in the back of the aircraft, with only just enough light to see the person next to you. We used the reflective belts we wore to determine where everyone else was sitting. An infantry soldier from Missouri sat directly across from me. His reflective belt shined and allowed just enough light to show the hand he had rested on his rifle. Sitting next to him was a girl name Melissa. She was from Arizona. Her blonde hair was pulled back into a bun, in order to comply with military hair dress regulations. She fidgeted back and forth, as if she was very uncomfortable.

Things were going well, until we entered into the city of Mosul, Iraq. By that point, I had been up for 24 hours and was exhausted from all the traveling. I managed to dose off to sleep, only to be awakened by loud sounds from outside the plane. I quickly looked around and everyone else also looked concerned. We heard more loud noises. Then it sounded like something ricocheted off the side of our plane, which seemed to resemble gunfire. I was correct. Our plane had been spotted, and we were taking enemy gunfire.

The plane carried the majority of our unit personnel, which ranged from doctors, nurses, respiratory therapists, critical care flight personnel, combat medics and infantry soldiers. It also carried most of our medical equipment. If our plane had been shot down, it would have been a tremendous loss to the Americans fighting the war against terrorism.

In southeast Asia, over 85% of all kills are attributed to an insurgent spotting and shooting the defender, without ever being seen. Still, even if we had spotted the person shooting at us, it would have been nearly impossible to return fire from the back of the C-130 aircraft. Our pilot had to make a quick decision or else 40-50 soldiers' lives would have been at risk.

All of a sudden, all lights on the plane turned off. The inside of the plane became even darker. The pilot yelled over the radio and told everyone to put their seat straps on. I could no longer see the soldier that had been sitting next to me. The pilot tilted the plane to the left, then to the right. The seat straps did not seem to help as I banged helmets with the soldier next to me. Each time the plane shifted directions, I was violently thrown from side to side. I tried to grab my plastic seat strap and brace myself from being thrown around, but that didn't seem to help either. Each time I regained my posture, I was thrown again as the pilot directed the nose of the plane in the opposite direction, trying to avoid being hit again by the insurgents.

Then suddenly, the engine of the plane turned off. We were then free falling through mid-air. All I could do at that point was pray. And pray I did – like I never had before.

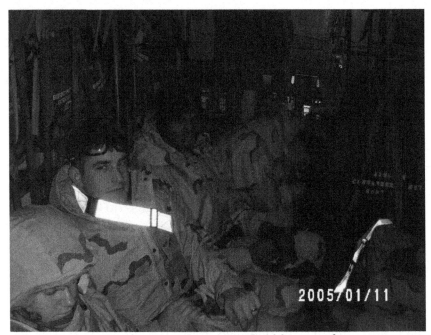

Heading into Iraq on a C-130 aircraft

The pilot attempted what is called a "combat landing" and thanks to his quick actions, we landed safely in Mosul. By that time, everyone was shook up but relieved to be safe on the ground. The back gate of the plane opened up and on the landing zone was a military ambulance. We were there to pick up three wounded soldiers whose Humvee had been ambushed a few hours earlier. The plan was to take them to our facility in Balad and then to Ramstein, Germany for further care.

Our goal in war, as medics, was to transport wounded troops out of the combat zone and get them to Germany, within 24 hours of injury. The first and most immediate care was battalion care, where a field medic administered initial aid to injured troops on the battlefield. The wounded soldiers were then taken to a combat support hospital, of which Balad was one, and then finally to Germany.

Landstuhl Regional Medical Center, in Ramstein Germany, was where wounded soldiers, from Iraq and Afghanistan, were taken for further care. From Germany, the wounded soldiers were flown back to the US and sent to either Walter Reed in Bethesda, Maryland or Brooke Army Medical Center in San Antonio, Texas.

BALAD, IRAQ

In late 2004, as the US invaded Fallujah, the Marines and Army secured multiple locations throughout Iraq and utilized those areas for various purposes. The areas were used as landing zones for planes, staging areas for equipment, living areas, and areas for providing medical care. An area, about 40 miles north of Baghdad, was secured in a small Shiite city called Balad. This area was then used as a location for our combat support hospital. By the time we arrived in Balad in January 2005, the tent hospital was already up and running, and accepting casualties.

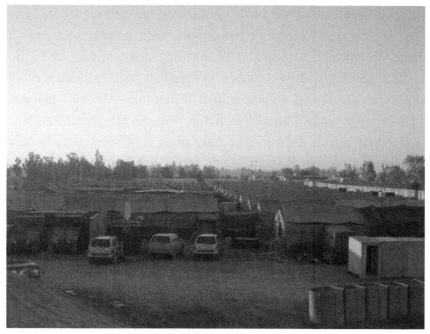

Our tent hospital

Balad was known as "Mortarville" for the frequency of rocket and missile attacks it received on a daily basis. It was said that about 80% of the attacks on coalition forces occurred in the Sunni triangle, which was formed by Baghdad, Tikrit, and Air Ramadi. Balad fell right in the middle of that zone. On average, we were attacked three to four times a day.

The military's intention was to create an environment, despite the dangerous war zone, that one would find similar to a small city back home in the United States. We first slept in large military tents and then transitioned to trailers, which we referred to as "hooches." The hooches were divided into three sections, each with its own door and a small triad of steps. Surrounding each hooch were five-foot high walls of dark green sandbags, which served as barriers to rockets and enemy gunfire. Inside, each hooch resembled the contents of a jail cell, but larger and without restrooms. The hooches contained a small bed, a lamp stand, and a mini cabinet to store our uniforms and combat gear.

To shower, we took a ten-minute walk to the "Cadillac"- a large white trailer equipped with showers, sinks, urinals, and toilet stalls. At times it seemed useless to take that walk and shower with our bullet proof vest on and helmet, when the walk back made us just as sweaty and fatigued as before the shower. Nonetheless, it was a safe haven for me - the only place that seemed to be kept genuinely clean by the base contractors. Each Cadillac contained a sign that read, "COMBAT SHOWERS IN EFFECT" which reminded soldiers to conserve water during war. We were given 30 seconds to get wet, and then 60 seconds to rinse off the lather.

On base, there was a Subway shop and a small Pizza Hut, which always seemed to have a long line. Saddam's old private pool was located nearby and had a 20-foot diving board, which we jumped from during our down time. There was also a movie theater called Sustainer, which once belonged to Saddam. The Sustainer was made out of marble and contained enough seats to sit 740 people. We often watched the latest movies, sometimes even before they hit theaters in the United States. Our gym consisted of large Alaskan tents that contained several exercise bikes and free weights. Soldiers from around the base often held weight lifting competitions at the gym. I reached a personal record of lifting 250 pounds on the bench press and was awarded a t-shirt for doing so.

To eat, we headed to the "DFAC"- short for dining facility. The DFACs were soft-sided tents and were run by base contractors. Meals were one of the few times that troops congregated in large groups and removed their bulletproof vest and helmets. Everyone knew the DFACs were prime target locations for the insurgents to attack, primarily because they could catch soldiers at one of their most vulnerable points and without protective gear. This allowed the insurgents to injure hundreds of troops at once. But, after wearing the 40-pound bulletproof vests for 8-10 hours straight, we looked forward to removing it so we could somewhat relax and enjoy our meal. That was just a risk we took.

Weeks before our arrival to Iraq, there was an insurgency attack at a DFAC in Mosul, Iraq. A member of the Iraqi insurgent group, Ansar al-Sunnah, walked into a DFAC and blew himself up. A powerful explosion tore through the mass tent. Twenty-two people were killed and 66 were wounded. Those killed and injured included Iraqi soldiers, civilian contractors, and US soldiers. The group that took responsibility for the bombing identified the bomber as Abu Omar of Mosul, and reported that he had slipped into the base through a hole in the fence during guard change. The bombing took place around the same time the military was building bunker-like dining areas to increase protection against mortar and rocket attacks. These bunkers were soon placed at various locations around the base, and we used them as barriers whenever the siren sounded to warn us of attacks. No matter where you were on base, it was a wise idea to know where the nearest bunker was, in case of an attack.

After every war in history, the lessons learned on the battlefield are utilized to improve the delivery of medical care during combat in future battles. Troops are constantly forced to come up with new ways to save lives. After World War I, forward aid stations and the use of blood transfusions on the battlefield were introduced. During World War II, thousands of soldiers were saved from deadly infections after the introduction and usage of the antibiotic penicillin. And, the Korean and Vietnam War paved the way for refined helicopter evacuation of injured troops and mobile surgical hospitals.

During World War I, the survival rate of wounded soldiers was 79%. During Operation Enduring Freedom, the survival rate increased to a remarkable 91%. This survival rate reached an astonishing 98% for troops who arrived at our combat hospital in Balad. This was because of the medical advances in technology, training, and innovation.

Every war has its signature weapon of choice. In Iraq, the weapons of choice were improvised explosive devices (IEDs) and landmines. IEDs presented battlefield challenges because they brought a chance of infection. They were often packed with shrapnel, such as dirty steel nuts and nails. Combined with bacteria from dirt, it made for a challenge to minimize infections. To alleviate the problem, wound debridements during combat were performed in our combat hospital to remove dead, damaged, and infected tissue. Negative pressure drainage devices were then applied to decrease swelling and retard further bacterial growth.

One of the most important innovations in war history, however, was the reemphasis of one of the oldest medical implements on the battlefield: tourniquets. These were issued in preparation for our deployment, with the understanding that they might be used to save each other's life. This turned out to be true when weeks later, the amputation rate in the Iraq war reached record highs. It was said that more than 1,270 Americans killed in combat during that time might have lived, if the military's emphasis on tourniquets had come sooner.

Before leaving the United States, we were trained on the proper set up and operation of our expeditionary medical facility – essentially our tent hospital. We spent a significant amount of time in the field running mock exercises and undergoing drills, where we simulated real combat scenarios. Instead of using real people or mannequins, we used live pigs as our patients. Pigs have similar vital statistics as humans, so we were able to evaluate the effectiveness of our interventions and pharmacologic treatments. Prior to the training, the pigs were anesthetized and traumatic injuries were inflicted on them. We were then tasked to quickly perform lifesaving interventions, such as placing breathing tubes, chest tubes, and intravenous lines. The pigs were hooked up to the cardiac monitor, which allowed us to see their blood pressure, heart rate, and oxygen saturation. At the end of our training, the pigs were euthanized.

Our EMEDS (Expeditionary Medical Support System) team was comprised of medical, administrative, and logistical troops. We were trained to deploy in a moment's notice, anywhere around the world. We had the capability to set up a fully functional medical facility within 24 hours. The basic premise of the set up was having a conglomerate of medical care modules that could be quickly assembled and transported to a battle site.

Various types of EMEDS teams existed. There was an EMEDS basic, EMEDS plus 10, and EMEDS plus 25. The EMEDS basic consisted of a two-person medical team and a five person mobile surgical team. Together, this formed a rapid response team that had the capacity to provide medical support to smaller combat situations.

In Balad, the EMEDS plus 25 team was activated, meaning our facility was set up to contain 25 beds and be run by more than 80 troops. Once it was set up, our tent hospital contained a triage area for quickly assessing soldiers, an ICU for critically ill patients, a ward for more stable patients, an operating room, a pharmacy, a radiology area where there was a mobile CT scanner, and a morgue.

Once we arrived in the country, we headed to the hospital to receive a tour. Medics, who were scheduled to leave not too long after we arrived, gave us a tour of the tent hospital and our living quarters. They were thrilled to see new, fresh faces and excited to finally be heading home after five long months of combat. During the tour, what I found most disturbing and hard to come to terms with, were the patient demographics on the wards.

The wards were located towards the back of the tent, which necessitated walking on the makeshift floors. The floors were made out of large sheets of wood and let out long *creeeeaks* as we walked over them. Inside the ward were twelve gurney combat stretchers, which were lined up on each side of the tent. Each one was filled with an injured patient. Above each stretcher were intravenous saline bags – for quick resuscitation, in the case a patient rapidly required fluids.

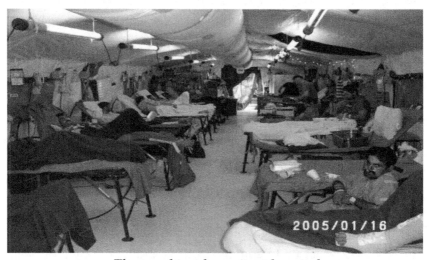

The ward inside our tent hospital

Some of the patients had been shot several times. Some had suffered traumatic brain injuries (TBIs) from hitting their heads as they were thrown onto the ground after the explosion. Some had blast and shrapnel injuries from improvised explosive devices (IEDs). What I quickly noticed, however, was how different all the patients seemed to be. Each gave me variable looks of despair and pain as I passed through the ward tent.

In the ward, next to a wounded soldier who was sleeping, was a gentleman handcuffed to his gurney. Two muscular American soldiers with large weapons sat on each side of him. They wore brown flak vests and military combat helmets. They looked at me and nodded their heads, then quickly looked away. I stole a quick glance at the gentleman who was between them. He appeared to be in pain. He constantly moved in bed, trying to find the best position, despite having his hands and feet chained down to the gurney.

"What is that Iraqi prisoner doing in this ward?" I asked.

"There is no separate place for the prisoners, so we keep them in here," stated one of the medics. He was scheduled to return to the US after we arrived.

"Right next to our Americans?" I asked in disbelief.

"Yes, unfortunately."

Something about that statement sent chills down my spine. I looked back at the prisoner, glanced at the American soldiers sitting on each side of him, and then shook my head in disbelief. I realized right away that having the Iraqi insurgent so close to our American soldiers could potentially present a problem during our deployment. Nonetheless, we continued on with the tour.

We headed back out into the main walkway of the tent, which connected the wards to the ICU upfront and the operating room in the back. The tent ceilings were no more than eight feet high. This required me to bend my 75-inch body frame down, as we passed by certain areas of the tent where the roof had collapsed, possibly from the heavy rain that occurred the night before. The inside of the tents were lined with vinyl to defend against dust and chemical attacks, important in an environment where infection and sterility were essential. Outside the tents were rows of port-o-potties, which were covered in mud. It had rained pretty hard the night before and the grounds had flooded, including the port-o-potties. Surrounding the hospital tent were hundreds of sandbags, piled high to minimize damage from rocket attacks. Even they had become saturated from the heavy rain.

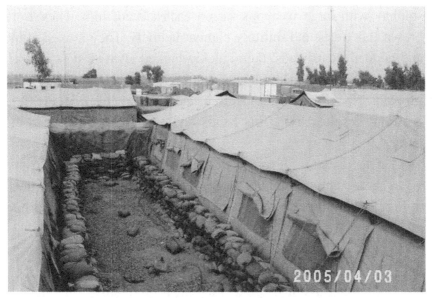

Hospital tent surrounded by sandbags

Also located outside the tents was the loading zone for the medevac Blackhawk. The loading zone was an area made out of concrete and it contained a big red cross in the center. In the middle of the night, the pilot used this cross as a landmark to land the chopper.

The loading zone was quickly utilized as our tour was abruptly halted by the sound of a chopper. It arrived to drop off several injured troops. Everyone stopped what they were doing and quickly moved to the triage area and landing zone. The rotors of the medevac chopped louder and louder as it approached, until the person I was talking to couldn't be heard anymore. The sound of chopper blades alerted everyone in the hospital that a trauma was en route, as several more medics met us by the loading zone. I crouched down and put earplugs in to minimize the noise of the chopper, then began to unload the wounded soldiers. Flight medics gave us a quick report of what happened.

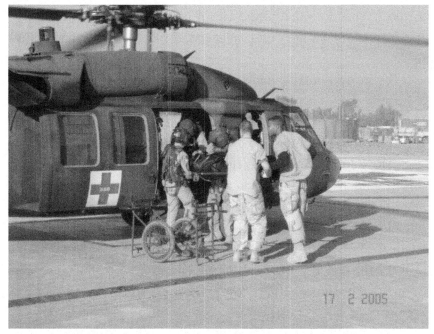

Transferring a wounded soldier off the medevac

"We have a 20-year-old soldier from Tikrit whose Humvee was ambushed by a group of insurgents. He has a gunshot wound over his left shoulder, which was dressed with a flutter valve, and shrapnel wounds to his face. His blood pressure is 105/67, heart rate 98, and oxygen saturation 94%"

I nodded, reassuring the flight medic that I understood his report and headed with the injured soldier to the front of our tents, where the triage area was located.

Each landing at the loading zone placed the flight medics and medevac pilots at risk of being shot down by the insurgents. The chopper quickly ascended back into the dusty air and flew to a nearby battlefield to retrieve more injured soldiers.

As I quickly assessed the injured soldier's wounds, a loud siren followed by a loud shout suddenly came over the intercom. "Alarm red! Alarm red!"

I looked around to see what was going on and asked a nearby medic, "What does that sound mean?"

"It means we are being attacked. Grab your gear and follow me."

We moved outside and quickly entered into a large barricade. It was the size of a small trailer, but was fortified with concrete for our protection. Inside the barricade were several seats. I quickly darted for the remaining one.

"How long do we have to stay in here?" I asked an Army medic who had already lit a cigarette and started smoking. He appeared to be well versed in being under attack, but was obviously frustrated by having to come into the barricade once again.

"Until we get the "all-clear" message on the intercom. Sometimes it can take only a few minutes, sometimes it can take hours."

Thankfully, that message did come a few minutes later. It wouldn't be too long after, that the realization truly sank in. *I was in war*.

A CLOSE CALL

In addition to providing medical care to injured troops, everyone was required to pull guard duty. Surrounding our hospital tents were several large, 10-foot high, concrete walls. Those walls were designed to minimize damage from rocket attacks by providing a barricade to our camp. However, the enemy was located just a hundred feet from the back of our tents. The only thing that separated our camp, from the enemy, was a wire fence. At the very least, all the enemy had to do was run up and toss a grenade over the fence. In an attempt to alleviate the chances of such a thing, snipers hid above our compound and looked down the scopes of their rifles for abnormal movement in the open land. They took out anyone who looked suspicious. But, often their vision was obscured…by sand storms.

Many times the sand storms were so bad that I couldn't see four feet in front of me. Outside, I wore a scarf to prevent sand from lodging down my throat, and on guard duty I wore goggles to prevent it from getting into my eyes. Some days the dust storms were so bad, aircrafts were restricted from flying. During those times, no patients could be flown in.

At the front of the hospital compound was the security checkpoint. Everyone who entered the hospital compound was required to present a military ID as they approached the checkpoint. That was followed by a thorough search of their vehicle to check for explosives and hidden weapons.

We rotated in eight-hour shifts. Many times, at night, I had to pull security duty alone. I found myself often reminiscing about life back in the US, while looking over my shoulder at every noise heard. Throughout my shift, I sometimes heard gunshots in the distance or loud explosions from mortars being shot towards our camp. Every explosion or gunfire I heard, I tried to gauge how far away it was by the loudness of the blast. I knew a mortar attack came *very* close to hitting me while on guard duty one evening. I reflexively curled up in a frenzy from the sounds of it detonating when it hit the ground. I then knew that injured patients would soon be pouring through our checkpoint to receive care.

Even though we were in a wartime situation, we still needed to gain the trust of the Iraqi people. We attempted this by providing free medical care to the Iraqis. We also went into the small villages of Balad and handed out humanitarian supplies and food. Most Iraqis did not want us in their country, however, which led to insurgency militants devising strategies to attack our camps.

On base, there were hundreds of contractors. They were hired by the government to run our DFACs, morale centers, and recreational facilities. At the hospital, several contractors were responsible for the cleaning and upkeep around our hospital tents. The insurgents soon picked up on this, and began hiring some of the contractors to obtain coordinates of our campgrounds. The coordinates were taken back and used for strategic and more precise RPG attacks on our camp. It wasn't until one contractor was caught with the layouts and coordinates of our camp that we began to catch on. They then needed other ways to infiltrate our camp. Soon, they began purposely injuring themselves by shooting themselves in the foot or stabbing themselves in the arm. They knew we would provide medical care for them at our facility. Once inside our facility, they observed what we were doing, the weapons we had, and how we operated on a day-to-day basis.

The more information they obtained about the layout and operation of our camp, the closer they came to hitting us with RPGs. This became evident during our second day in country.

Ali was the name of one of my patients. He was an Iraqi civilian, who suffered traumatic extremity injuries after insurgents attacked his house with bombs.

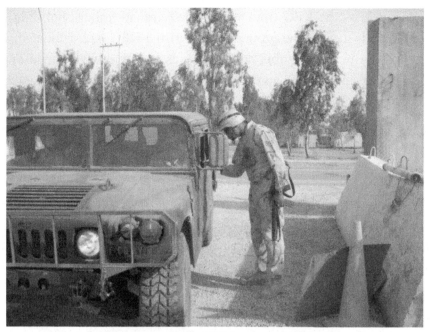

Guard duty with M-16 weapon in hand

He unfortunately lost several family members during the bombing, and began to voice his frustration about the war and how he did not like the Americans being in his country. The frustration could be heard through his candidly broken English voice. However, when he was in pain, he spoke in Arabic. "Alam, alam!" became an Arabic word I'd never forget.

While changing his dressing, I heard a big *swoosh* go right over my head. This was immediately followed by a big thud as an object hit the ground. I looked around and no one said a word. Some people reached for their gear while others stood still, in shock. Then the loud sirens came on. This was followed by an overhead announcement stating that we had been attacked. I grabbed and donned my helmet and Kevlar vest. I then tried to locate my troops, to make sure they were ok. The insurgents acquired our coordinates and were getting very close to hitting our camp, this time within feet from where I was standing.

Luckily, the RPG (rocket propelled grenade) they shot didn't explode. It just hit the ground, a dud. If the RPG had detonated, I would not be writing this book today as it would have wiped out our entire camp. A group of Air Force troops, called the Explosive Ordinance Team, arrived to complete and remove the live explosive. Minutes later, a soldier yelled through the radio, "The target has been extinguished." We knew then that the person who shot the rocket was killed. After hearing this, I took off my bulletproof vest and helmet, and headed back inside the hospital. I couldn't help but think that I could have been killed or injured that day, but I was incredibly relieved and thankful that I was unharmed. And it was only *day two*. We now had a battle on our hands.

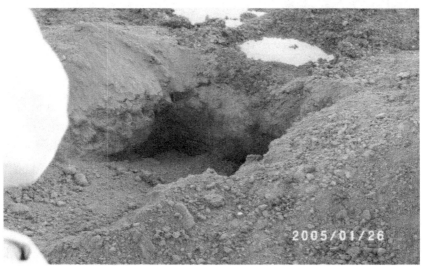

Hole made by the RPG that landed right outside our hospital tent

MASS CASUALTY

Feb 13, 2005 3:40am: We received word that several injured patients were being flown in to our hospital from Baghdad. In combat, we called this a MASCAL (mass casualty). This occurred when the number of injured patients exceeded the available medical capability to rapidly treat and evacuate them. When this occurred, we activated our emergency response system to alert everyone to report to the hospital for additional manpower. Some medics helped by unloading the wounded soldiers off the chopper, while others assisted in searching the patients for weapons or explosive devices. The remaining soldiers triaged patients as they came in.

Effective mass casualty response is founded on the principle of triage — the system of sorting and prioritizing injured patients based on the extent of their injuries and available resources. During a mass casualty, in a peacetime environment, the sickest patients are treated first. The more stable patients are treated last. In war, it's just the opposite. When several injured soldiers came in at once, a quick triage was performed. Care was provided to the most stable patient first — with the idea to get the most warfighters back to fighting, as quickly as possible.

During our triages, the injured patients were placed in categories of immediate, delayed, minimal or expectant. Patients who were placed in the immediate category had life-threatening injuries that required immediate action. They had a reasonable chance at survival. These injuries included gunshot wounds, multiple extremity amputations, and severe burns. Soldiers in this category were tended to quickly and given red tags. Soldiers who came in with non-survivable injuries, in comas, or deceased were placed in the expectant category and given a black tag. Their injuries were so severe that we didn't have the resources or manpower to provide them with adequate care. The more stable soldiers were called the "walking wounded." They required medical care at some point, but not right away. They were given green tags, patched up, and sent back out to fight.

Before leaving to Iraq, we received extensive training on how to respond if and when this happened. It wouldn't be long before our preparedness was put to the test.

Coming back from a night patrol, several Army soldiers were in a military Humvee when their truck flipped over and rolled off in a canal. Three soldiers were killed instantly. Five additional soldiers were sent to our hospital. Once they arrived, we quickly triaged them and discovered that they only had minor injuries. They were all given green tags and eventually went back out to the battlefield. Unfortunately, I can't say the same for everyone that evening.

A firefighter, from San Antonio and deployed with the 7th Civil Engineering Squadron, would be the first casualty during our deployment. As part of the rescue mission, Sergeant Wood was the first person to jump in the water to help save the drowning soldiers. The strong current of the river quickly swept him away. He disappeared in the waves and his body was later found downstream. Sergeant Wood's death really hit home. He was from our hometown and died while trying to save others. He left behind a wife and three children.

Minutes later, a Blackhawk landed with four wounded National Guard soldiers with gunshot and shrapnel wounds.

The chopper had just flown in from Tikrit, Iraq after an intense six-hour battle with insurgents. Two soldiers died in the firefight. There was no landing zone where the soldiers were picked up in the middle of the battle. Soldiers on the ground had to throw purple smoke grenades to let the pilot know where to land amongst the heavy desert dust.

The chopper quickly descended to our landing zone. We stood back behind a tall concrete barricade to minimize being caught amongst the sand storm that was created by the rotating chopper blades. We then donned our goggles to prevent the sand from getting into our eyes. Once on the ground, the flight medic waved and signaled at us to approach the chopper.

The first gurney was unloaded from the chopper by two flight medics. One hand of each soldier held onto the gurney. The other hand held onto the trigger of their M-16 weapon, ready to fire at a moment's notice. According to the Geneva conventions, military medical personnel are not allowed to fire their weapons while providing medical care. Similarly, enemy insurgents are not allowed to fire upon vehicles or medical personnel displaying the Red Cross. Nonetheless, this was war and during war, anything goes. Even though the Blackhawk had white decals with a red cross on the sides, and rules of war prohibited firing on medical vehicles, the soldiers did not want to take any chances.

After handoff, we rushed the first injured soldier to the triage area and quickly assessed his wounds. Blood dripped and soaked through the green gurney as he moaned in pain.

"I think I shot a kid, I think I shot a kid," the soldier screamed.

"What happened, man? Why do you think that?" I asked.

I attempted to calm him down by starting a conversation. I then used my trauma shears to cut off his bloody camouflage cargo trousers to evaluate his injuries. Another medic attempted to place a fourteen gauge IV into his vein.

"We ran into the house and the next thing I know, someone from nowhere started shooting. I think I shot a little kid when I fired back. I just want to get back out there with my soldiers."

Even though he was injured, he was most upset about leaving his fellow troops behind. He wanted to get back out there and fight – an attitude shared by every soldier I treated while there.

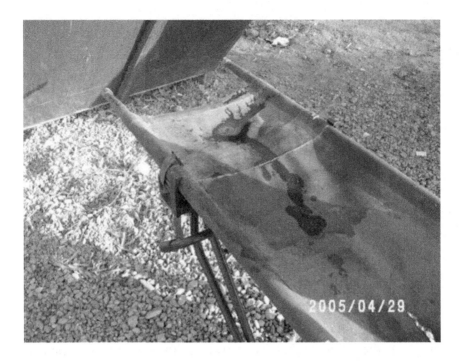

2005/04/29

I quickly bandaged him up, gave him something for pain through his IV, and ran back to the landing zone to retrieve the rest of the injured soldiers.

We repeated that grueling process several more times that day and had numerous more MASCALS during the remainder of my deployment. Each time, we received several injured soldiers at once, ranging from gunshot injuries to mangled extremity amputation wounds. And, each time we worked hard to save as many lives as we could. Our goal was to stabilize injured patients, minimize the number of black body bags that were being filled, and get them to Germany as quickly as possible. Our role in this process, as medics, would turn out to be vital during the war. Our tireless efforts, to meet our transport time of moving injured troops out of the combat zone within 24 hours and safely to Germany, helped achieve "the lowest mortality rate ever seen in modern warfare."

DIFFICULT TRANSITION

I took care of 800+ patients during my time in Iraq. I also earned several medals for my service including: an Air Force Achievement medal, Meritorious Unit Award medal, National Defense Service medal, Iraq Campaign Ribbon, Global War on Terrorism Service medal, and an Air Force Expeditionary Service Ribbon. It is safe to assume that all soldiers are impacted by war, whether psychologically or physically.

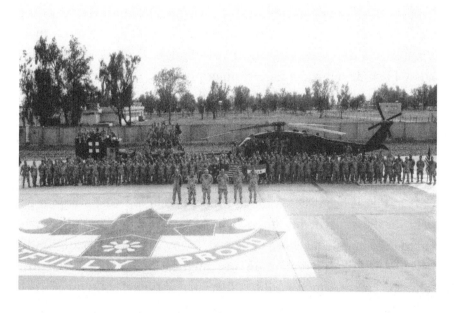

Returning home from war was a difficult transition for me. Upon leaving Iraq, my unit met with behavioral health individuals who administered PTSD (post-traumatic stress disorder) screening questionnaires. One of the drawbacks of being in the military and around your fellow troops is that "no one wants to talk about it." That is, being affected by going to war. The general rule was to keep quiet. If you were having problems, you had better not said anything. Promotions, respect from fellow colleagues, and the thought of being ostracized kept a lot of my fellow troops, including myself, quiet. So, when the questionnaire hit my desk and I was asked, "Are you having trouble sleeping?" "Do loud noises startle you?" "Do you have nightmares?" I quickly answered no, even though I was experiencing all of the above.

Returning to the states, around the July 4th holiday, made it difficult to be outside. The loud noises from the fireworks and the sight of projectile explosions from firecrackers immediately gave me vivid flashbacks. I often woke up in the middle of the night thinking about the explosions I heard, the deaths that occurred, and the gruesome injuries I had seen. Still, I didn't talk about it. I just kept quiet. When people confronted me and asked me if everything was ok, I blew them off. My response was usually, "I'm ok man. I'm just a little stressed out." Even though, deep down inside, I knew I had developed a raging anger problem.

Before leaving to Iraq, I had only gotten into one fight. And that was when I was a younger kid – much younger, in fact. Post deployment, I found the war zone had turned me into a furious fighting animal. Within the first year, I got into four fistfights. I often lost my temper quickly and in a moment's notice. So quickly, in fact, that it even scared me at times. I contemplated going to get help. In the back of my mind though, I knew seeking help meant having my medical record "flagged." Any diagnosis made by the psychiatrist would remain in my medical record for my entire military career, and would affect my future deployments and promotions. I didn't want to be labeled as someone who "had an appointment with the psychiatrist." I continued to keep it to myself, until it eventually lead to my arrest.

One evening while out with friends, I got into an altercation with another guy. The event resulted in my arrest, a misdemeanor charge, a mandatory anger management class, and thousands of dollars in fines, court costs, and lawyer fees. It was then that I realized the need for professional help. I made an appointment at the VA Mental Health Clinic to be seen. After a workup, I was diagnosed with a mild form of PTSD.

Even to this day, some ten years later, I still have flashbacks of what I saw while I was deployed. Whenever I hear a loud noise, or even just a door slamming, I'm immediately reminded of the rockets that were fired and the explosions of missiles hitting the ground. I've noticed that whenever I sit at a table, such as in a restaurant or classroom, I tend to not sit with my back towards the door. I have to be facing the door so that I can see who is coming in and who is leaving. I never had that problem before going to Iraq. They say it gets better with time, but it's been almost ten years and I still have residual symptoms of PTSD from the war.

The phenomenon is all too common these days. Soldiers return straight home after spending 6-12 months under fire every day, most likely taking the lives of others in the process. And when they return home, they are expected to act, think, and behave normally again. Instead, once they arrive home, alcohol abuse, traffic accidents, and other events arise as soldiers blow off steam.

I once heard the story of a soldier who returned home from a nine-month deployment from Iraq. Upon his return, he felt like everything and everyone had changed, so he went off on a shooting spree and killed several people in the process. There was also the story of Sgt. Daniel Somer, an Iraq war veteran, who took his life in 2013. He left behind a powerful suicide note, which went viral on the Internet, after his family shared it with media. In it, he stated, "My body has become nothing but a cage, a source of pain and constant problems. The illness I have has caused me pain that not even the strongest medicines could dull, and there is no cure." Somers went on to write, "All day, every day, a screaming agony in every nerve ending in my body. It is nothing short of torture. My mind is a wasteland, filled with visions of incredible horror, unceasing depression, and crippling anxiety."

Soon after, the VA released information showing that 22 military veterans commit suicide every day. This prompted the

Obama administration to allocate more funding for veterans and sign an order to improve veteran and service member access to mental health screenings.

ADVICE:

Post-traumatic stress disorder (PTSD) is a mental health condition that is triggered by a terrifying event – either experiencing it or witnessing it. After a trauma, car accident, or life-threatening event such as sexual or physical abuse, it is common to have deep psychological reactions. Some potential reactions include: upsetting memories of the event, trouble sleeping, nightmares, severe anxiety, increased likelihood of being startled, or flashbacks. These can cause significant problems in social or work situations, and in relationships. Most people who experience traumatic events have difficulty coping for a while, but with good self-care and support they usually get better. If the reactions do not get better or go away, or if they get worse, you may have PTSD.

PTSD symptoms are generally grouped in four types: intrusive memories, avoidance, changes in emotional reactions, and negative changes in thinking and mood.

Symptoms of intrusive memories:
- Recurrent, unwanted, upsetting memories of the traumatic event
- Reliving the traumatic event as if it were happening again (flashbacks)
- Distressing dreams about the traumatic event

Symptoms of avoidance:
- Trying to avoid thinking or talking about the traumatic event
- Avoiding people, places or activities that remind you of the traumatic event

Symptoms of negative changes in thinking and mood:
- Negative feelings about yourself or other people
- Inability to experience positive emotions
- Feeling emotionally numb
- Lack of interest in activities you once enjoyed
- Hopelessness about the future
- Memory problems, including not remembering important aspects of the traumatic event
- Difficulty maintaining close relationships

Symptoms of changes in emotional reactions:
- Irritability, angry outbursts, or aggressive behavior
- Always being on guard for danger
- Overwhelming guilt or shame
- Self-destructive behavior, such as drinking too much or driving too fast
- Trouble concentrating
- Trouble sleeping
- Being easily startled or frightened

When to see a doctor?
- If you have disturbing thoughts and feelings about a traumatic event for greater than a month
- If you are having trouble getting back to your normal life
- If you have thoughts of hurting yourself

If you are in a crisis, you DO have options:
- Reach out to a close friend or loved one
- Contact a minister or spiritual leader
- Call 911
- Go to the nearest Emergency Room
- Call the suicide prevention lifeline 1-800-273-TALK (273-8255)

Recognize the signs of PTSD and GET HELP! Don't wait until it's almost too late - like I did. By the time I was arrested, it was already too late. The damage had already occurred. As a result, I suffered the consequences when I later applied to medical school.

PATH TO SUCCESS

As a Combat Medic in the U.S. Air Force, I bore many obligations and responsibilities. While on active duty, I somehow still managed to attend evening, internet, and even weekend courses to continue working towards my goals of becoming a physician.

A few months after arriving at my first duty station, Lackland Air Force base in San Antonio, Texas, I enrolled at a local community college named St. Phillips College. The advantage of starting off at a community two-year college is two-fold. First, it is cheaper than attending a four-year university. This saves thousands of dollars in tuition and in fees. Secondly, classes are usually smaller. This can be beneficial because of the opportunity to receive more face time with professors, and they in turn, can get to know you better.

During that first semester, my schedule with the military only allowed me to take classes at night and on the weekends. I signed up for two classes, English 101 and History 101.

"Your first paper is due next week, please let me know if you have any questions."

My professor didn't know that I was in the military, nor did she know that I was studying to become a doctor. I had written papers in high school, and was pushed academically by one of my high school senior teachers to prepare for college. But, for some reason, I was nervous about writing the two-page paper. I rushed home, swerving through rush hour traffic, and headed straight to my black Dell desktop computer. Eight words later, tears began to flow down my face. I just couldn't come up with the words to write. Writer's block hit me hard. My goal of becoming a doctor flashed before my eyes and I contemplated giving up.

It's too much work. I can never do this, I thought.

After what felt like ages of frustration, something told me to just take a nap and try again when I woke up. I quickly exited my computer and went straight to my bed. Two hours later, I woke up and successfully wrote my paper.

My first English paper assignment was, by no means, the most challenging part of my undergraduate career. That turned out to be attending school full time while serving on active duty Air Force. I typically worked 40-50 hours a week, in addition to a part time job. This forced me to attend five different schools during the six-year span of completing my undergraduate degree. I attended classes whenever and wherever I could. Several times, I was forced to drop classes because of military obligations, but thankfully my professors were all very understanding.

When I worked the day shift at the military hospital, I went to school at night or took internet courses. I often came home late and slept for only a few hours before doing it again the next day. When I worked the night shift in the ICU, I left work at 7:00 am, after working a 12-hour shift, and attended class from 8:00 am-2:00 pm. I rushed home to shower, eat, and sleep until I woke up for work at 5:00 pm. I repeated that grueling process for several years. I feel it's safe to say that those six years were the most exhausting years of my life. But, what I didn't know was that those years would ultimately prepare me for the most challenging ones of my life: medical school.

ADVICE:

What are you willing to sacrifice in order to reach your goals? When I came home from work in the military and my friends wanted to hang out, I had to politely decline their offers. I had to miss a lot of parties, hangouts, and meet-ups with friends in order to focus on my studies. Sometimes when we think of the word 'sacrifice', we think of completely selfless acts in which one person does something for someone else. This reminds me of my time in Iraq when infantry soldiers sacrificed and put their lives on the line for our country. But, sacrifice isn't always solely altruistic. The law of sacrifice states you cannot get something you want, without giving up something in return. In order to obtain something, which you believe is of greater value, you must give up something you believe is of lesser value.

The times I decided to hit the books and study, instead of hanging out with my friends, meant that I was giving up something which I thought was of lesser value (partying) for something which I thought was of greater value (my education). Yes, my friends talked about me and called me names. But, looking back I have no regrets.

In life, believe it or not, we all make sacrifices. Whether we are making the right sacrifices is the question. Going out to a party and staying out until 2:00 am or 3:00 am means you are sacrificing sleep and most likely sacrificing money. Watching your favorite TV show means you are sacrificing time spent doing something more productive. To reach your ultimate goals and dreams in life, you must move forward. This requires making sacrifices and leaving some things behind.

Sacrifices=Success

How bad do you want it? Are you willing to do whatever it takes to achieve your goal? Are you willing to sacrifice friends, family, money, and prestige for a short time in order to achieve a long-term gain? Are you willing to stay up all night to prepare for your exam or big presentation the next day? Believe it or not, most people are not willing to do this. There is a quote that states, "Do the work others aren't willing to do and you'll get the things others will never have." Was I tired when I worked 50-60 hours a week in the military? Of course! I was extremely tired and exhausted when I got off of work. I could have gone home and slept, kicked back, and hung out with my friends. But I was willing to sacrifice those things for a greater gain – my education and future.

I once heard a story about Kobe Bryant, who is arguably one of the most successful players in basketball. He is a 5x NBA champion, 2x NBA finals MVP, and the Los Angeles Lakers all-time leading scorer.

The story went like this: It was about 3:30 am and one of Kobe's trainers was in his bed about to dose off to sleep when his phone rang. It was Kobe Bryant.

"Hey, uhh Mark I hope I am not disturbing anything right now," Kobe stated.

"No, not at all. What's up Kobe?"

"I was just wondering if you could just help me out with some conditioning work, that's all," Kobe stated.

Mark checked his clock and it was 3:35am.

"Yeah, sure I will be right there. I will meet you at the gym."

When the trainer finally arrived, he saw Kobe alone in the gym, drenched in sweat. He had already taken a swim, worked out, shot several hundred shots, and did some weights. And, it was only 4:30am.

Why would someone as successful as Kobe Bryant be up at 3:30 am in the morning and at the gym working out? Dedication! Doing things that others aren't willing to do, in order to be successful. To be successful, this is what you will have to do. No one will become successful by sleeping in until 10:00 am or 11:00 am. No one will be successful by putting in 50% effort. No one will be successful by doing things that everyone else is doing, just to get by.

Motivational speaker Eric Thomas nailed it when he said, "When you want to succeed as bad as you want to breathe, then you will be successful." He related this to an asthmatic patient. When someone has an asthma attack, it can be quite frightening for them. Sometimes, asthma attacks can lead to death. When asthmatics can't breathe, they don't worry about anything else. They don't worry about what is on TV, about which club will be the most packed that night, or about which new movie is at the theater. All they are concerned about is catching that next fresh breath of air. I'm not sure if you have ever been short of breath, but believe me, it is scary.

When I was younger, I wasn't paying attention and walked too far out in the pool while swimming. I didn't realize that the pool became deeper the farther I went out. I was playing in the water one second, and the next second, I was head deep under water. I almost drowned. I panicked and gasped for air. At that moment, I wasn't worried about what my friends were doing. I wasn't worried about who had the biggest rims. I wasn't worried about what was on TV. The only thing I was worried about was catching my next breath of air. When you want to be successful, as bad as gasping for your next breath of air, then you will be successful.

So, how bad do you want it?

Here are five things successful people are more willing to do:

- *They go to work to prosper, not just to work.* Those who are most successful go to work to accomplish something. They don't just go to work to "clock hours." They put in the hours and make time to perfect their craft, whether this means staying later or arriving early, before everyone else. Kobe Bryant could easily at this point in his career just show up to games and not put in hours of practice to perfect his craft. Instead, he wants to be successful. In order to do that, he put in the hours. A plastic surgeon once told me, "If you want to be a great surgeon and learn to suture skin well, get some sutures and practice tying surgical knots on your steering wheel at every red light." I gave him a confused look at first, and then realized he was right. To be successful, you have to do things other people aren't willing to do. That was the most brilliant thing I had heard that day. The most successful surgeons I know have done similar things to perfect their craft.

- *They exercise incredible drive.* The most successful people I know have extraordinary ambition, are focused, and never quit until the job is done. They keep doing the hard things while others are only doing what is comfortable to them. They go above and beyond what is required of them, and are always looking for ways for improvement.

- *They never make excuses.* Successful people know that making excuses will not change the outcome. When things go astray, successful people see it as an opportunity, not an insurmountable obstacle. When these excuses arise, listen to them and understand why you have them. They will only slow you down.

> *"No one ever excused their way to success."*
> Dave Del Dotto

- *They focus on their goals daily.* Successful people are always focused on success. They write down their goals and speak them into existence. Writing your goals down serves several purposes. First, it forces you to clarify what you want. Secondly, It forces you to select something specific and formulate a plan to make it happen. Every dream or goal will encounter resistance and the fear of failure. From the very moment you first write it down, you will feel it. Writing allows you to face this resistance head on, and the opportunity to tackle it strategically.

- *They are willing to take risks.* Successful people are willing to take risks when others aren't. They strive for these opportunities and know that if they don't put themselves in a position to fail, they'll never have an opportunity to win.

GOD WORKS IN MYSTERIOUS WAYS

While walking home from a long day of lectures one evening, I began to reminisce on the path that I had to take to get where I was in life. During those thoughts, I remembered back to 2004, when I initially started the process of applying to medical school. It was then that I began to wonder, and didn't know whether I should put in all the hard work, dedication and commitment that would be required to become a physician. I heard horror stories about individuals trying many years to get into medical school and once getting in, about how hard and challenging it was. I also knew that historically, I wasn't a good standardized test taker and medical school was extremely competitive with a required high MCAT (Medical College Admission Test) score. It was always a dream of mine to become a physician since high school but I somehow started doubting myself, becoming somewhat complacent. I then decided that medical school would be far-fetched, would cost too much money and the schooling would be too long. So instead, I decided to apply to PA (Physician Assistant) school.

Physician Assistants work under the supervision of a medical physician and are trained to examine patients, diagnose injuries and provide treatment. I took my SAT's, which were required, acquired all of my letters of recommendations, shadowed a PA for a couple of months, and made sure I had all the required courses so that I could apply. I was certain that this was what I wanted to do and could not wait to start PA school. A couple of weeks later after the PA acceptance board had met, I received a letter in the mail.

The results for acceptances came out and guess what, I was REJECTED.

That was probably one of the hardest failures that I had to face. I began to question myself and asked myself, *where did I go wrong? What could I have done differently? Am I not smart enough to do this?* All of these questions ran through my head, as I was sure that I would have at least gotten a standby acceptance. I recollected myself and kept taking classes here and there for the next one to two years. I prayed about it and talked to friends and family, majority of them encouraging me to go ahead and apply to medical school. Others told me I wouldn't have a chance, because of my grades, MCAT score, and arrest history.

Before applying to medical school, one has to take the pre-requisites (usually in courses such as General Chemistry, Organic Chemistry, Physics, and Biology), obtain letters of recommendation and to be competitive, spend hours shadowing and volunteering. The application process can be quite expensive, ranging anywhere from $1,000-$5,000 on fees, flights to interviews and hotels. In addition, matriculating into any medical school at all is competitive to say the least. The Association of American Medical Colleges' reported that more than 56 percent of medical school applicants were rejected in 2008. Knowing this, I knew my best odds would be to apply early and apply broadly.

From 2008 until 2010, I applied to medical school. Every day, I patiently checked my email, praying for just one school to give me a chance. A few interviews came in, but year after year more rejections rolled in. After interviewing at one particular school, I received this email:

Good Morning Antonio,

Our committee reviewed your application yesterday and, unfortunately, determined not to proceed with your candidacy for the Class of 2008. This decision was based on the committee's belief that you are not a good fit for our institution. I apologize I am unable to provide additional information regarding their reasoning.

Please know we wish you only the best.

Sincerely,

XXXXX

Every few days, I received a similar email but each worded a little differently. However, all intended to relay the same message, "You are competitive to apply, but not competitive enough to matriculate." What was most hurtful to me was that the school that sent the above email had invited me for an interview but I couldn't figure out why, "I wasn't a good fit for their institution." I felt pretty good after leaving the interview and bonded well with my interviewers. They were impressed with my background and seemed interested in having me as a student at their school. I am not sure what went wrong. I took that year's slew of rejections harder than the year prior. When I finally came to terms and accepted the fact that I would not be going to medical school after two straight years of applying, I broke down in tears. I thought of myself as a failure at that point. I contemplated quitting all together but something deep down inside of me kept telling me otherwise. I got on the phone with my advisor, gave him the bad news, and went back to the drawing board.

I had just gotten out of the military in 2009 and landed a job as a LVN (Licensed Vocational Nurse) in the ICU at Wilford Hall Medical Center in San Antonio, Texas. Our military medical training as medical technicians and EMT-B's (Emergency Medical Technician-Basic) allowed us to "test out" of the California LVN program. I studied for a few months for the exam, took it and became LVN certified. Once I found out I wasn't going to medical school and would have to reapply, I knew my best option would be to focus on my MCAT. The MCAT is an 8-hour standardized, multiple-choice exam designed to assess problem solving, critical thinking skills, knowledge of science concepts and principles. It is a prerequisite to medical school matriculation. Scores are reported in Physical Sciences, Verbal Reasoning, and Biological Sciences. These scores are added to give you a total score. Almost all U.S. medical schools and many Canadian schools require applicants to submit MCAT exam scores before applying. By that point, I had taken the MCAT twice and each time, I scored under the national mean. I figured the best way to get into medical school was to retake it and aim for a higher score. I also knew if I didn't have to work at the ICU, I would have more time to focus on my studies. It was a hard decision to quit because my job in the ICU was my only source of income. But, I knew I needed to sacrifice something in order to provide me the best opportunity to do well on the exam. I put in my two-week notice and quit my job at the ICU. Not having any income coming in, I needed another source of income. I ended up starting my own business, which I ran successfully for the next 6-12 months while studying full time for the MCAT.

One year later, it was time to apply for medical school again for the third time. I prayed, meditated and then submitted my application. During the application process, I searched and came across a program called the Georgetown Experimental Medical Studies Program (GEMS). The GEMS program is a one year post baccalaureate program designed for students from disadvantaged backgrounds who are most likely to make a significant contribution to meeting the needs of the nation's minority, disadvantaged and under-served populations, and whose disadvantaged circumstances have contributed to modest academic credentials. By the time medical school would have started, I would have not have set foot in a classroom or reviewed any science in over two years. I figured that a program like GEMs would prepare me academically for medical school, even though it would require me to do an additional year of schooling. I also knew that applying would be a long shot, given that the acceptance rates were very low and how competitive and stringent the screening process was. To my surprise, I was invited for an interview. Weeks later, I received a large brown envelope in the mail. This single brown envelope would forever change my life and would contain my acceptance letter to the GEMS program and Georgetown University. When others schools closed the door on my goals of becoming a physician, Georgetown took a chance and gave me an opportunity. I will be forever grateful. This program ultimately changed the way I studied, took exams and essentially set me up for success in medical school. I successfully completed the grueling one-year program and received acceptance into Georgetown University School of Medicine on May 28, 2010 at 10:53am. I consider that day one of the greatest days of my life.

Thinking back, one of my deans and mentor at Georgetown once stated, "Failure is not in the falling down, it is in the failing to get back up and try again." His statement really drove home an excellent point as I viewed myself as a failure at several points in my life. But, what I didn't know was that God had a GREATER plan for my life. I sometimes just sit back and ponder. If I would have been accepted to PA school in 2004, or if I would have gave up on applying to medical school all together after getting rejected the first or even the second time around, I most likely would of ended my education there. I also would not have become a physician and surgeon. Revelation 3:8 states, "The Lord will open doors that no man can close, and close doors that no man can open."

So, remember this verse when you are faced with obstacles in life, confronted with the odds or when it seems that every door is being closed on your dreams and goals. Keep praying during these times, stay patient, and don't give up. God will eventually open the door!

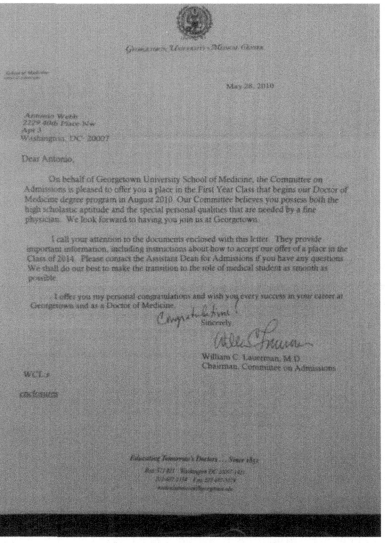

Medical School Acceptance Letter

ADVICE:

Failure is normal. Expect it. Learn from it. Not everyone likes to talk about it, which makes it look like they never fail, but don't fall for this trap.

Michael Jordan is arguably the greatest and most successful player to ever play the game of basketball. Maybe even the greatest athlete, regardless of sport. Why? Because he was a master of failure. He faced it over and over in life. And, he succeeded because of how he reacted to those failures. When he played JV basketball in high school, Michael Jordan was cut from the team. He could have given up right then and quit. He could have left that gym and never touched a basketball again. But what did he do? He learned from it, went back to the drawing board, worked harder, and went on to become one of the greatest athletes to ever live.

When you are faced with failure or presented with obstacles in life, don't let it stop you. When you run into these walls, don't turn around or give up. Figure out a way to climb it, go through it, or work around it. Michael Jordan once stated, "I've missed more than 9000 shots in my career. I've lost almost 300 games. Twenty-six times, I've been trusted to take the game winning shot and missed. I've failed over and over and over again in my life. And that is why I succeed."

How many shots in life are you willing to take before you give up? Or, you can be like many other successful people who succeeded but faced failure initially. For example, there is Steven Spielberg who was denied by USC's prestigious film school not once, but twice. He went on to become one of the most wealthiest and successful filmmakers in history. In 1994, USC named him an honorary alumnus and dedicated a building to him. Or there is Walt Disney, who was fired by a newspaper editor because, "he lacked imagination and had no good ideas." He then went on to start a number of businesses that didn't last long, ending in bankruptcy and failure. He didn't let this stop him. Instead he kept plugging along, eventually forming a billion dollar empire — Disneyland.

What does the Bible say about failure? Philippians 4:13 says, "I can do all things through Christ which strengthens me." To fail from time to time is only human, but to be a "failure" is when we are defeated by failure, refusing to rise and try again. Christians often believe they should be immune to failure by virtue of their relationship with God, but the truth is that God often allows us to fail for a variety of reasons. Job 14:1 says, "Man born of woman is of few days and full of trouble." That doesn't say "unbelievers" or "the ungodly." It says man born of woman. What does that mean? Everyone! Life is full of trouble, even for those who belong to God through faith in Christ. We are to expect it. This means God does not promise life to be without problems, sorrow, and yes, failure just because we believe in him.

Luke 9:1-5 describes how Jesus sent his disciples out to preach the gospel and perform miracles. He also taught them how to handle failure. "If people do not welcome you, shake the dust off your feet when you leave their town, as a testimony against them." Jesus wanted the soon-to-be apostles to model themselves after him. He gave them power and authority over devils, and power to heal the sick. Most of all, Jesus wanted them to have boldness. He knew that not everyone was going to receive the truth about him but in saying, "Shake the dust from your feet," he meant to move on and plow forward. Witnessing and being rejected can make us feel like failures, but if we understand we are to expect it (John 15:18), what appears to be failure actually becomes a badge of honor.

SECTION III:
MEDICINE

FROM MORTARVILLE TO MEDICAL SCHOOL

The first two years of medical school are spent in the classroom, learning the basic sciences of medicine. During my first year of medical school, we took classes such as Biochemistry, Molecular and Cellular Physiology, Genetics, Nutrition, Embryology, Histology, and Anatomy of the whole body. It was a very complex, fast paced year that was equivalent to 100+ hours of college credit.

When I gave a speech to 30+ high school students from Seneca Valley High School in Maryland, I compared the transition from high school to medical school using sports. I told them that high school academics was like playing on a varsity basketball team. A lot of people are good and some people are not so good. But, in all, you have some talented players and some people who just don't belong on the team. Compare this to high school academics – it's not really that hard. You basically show up, study a little bit and then move on to college. I told them in college basketball, players are usually bigger, quicker and stronger. Compare this to academics – students in college are usually smarter, classes are more intense, and a lot more work and studying is required. Medical school is like the NBA; everyone is quick, skilled, and professionals at what they do. Likewise, everyone in your medical school class is intelligent, professional, and bright. In addition, there is a lot more work along with a challenging atmosphere.

I discovered early in my first year that I learned best and was more efficient studying at home. So, I never attended class unless it was mandatory. My schedule varied by the day, but usually went as follows: woke up at 6:00 am to read or do practice questions until 10:00 am, studied from 10:00 am-5:00 pm, worked out at

6:00 pm, and then came home to study again from 8:00 pm-11:00 pm. During my first year of medical school, I definitely stayed up later to study. Sometimes this was until 3:00 am. As the years went on, I became more efficient with my time and more comfortable with studying less. Taking so many exams in medical school, I learned to read through 100+ pages of notes and pick out what was important to know for the exam and what were minutia details. Developing that skill definitely came handy during second year when I was expected to know twice as much information, in a shorter amount of time.

A unique component of our education at Georgetown was early clinical exposure. Day one of medical school, we started seeing and interviewing patients in the hospital. One day during my first year, I decided to take a break from studying and strolled over to the Georgetown Emergency Room. I wanted to see a few patients and put what I was learning in the classroom into a clinical setting picture. Within the first 30 minutes of working, I saw a patient with a rotator cuff injury and another one with Sickle Cell Anemia (SCA). I spent some time talking to the parent of the Sickle Cell Anemia patient, and made sure to check on her frequently between seeing other patients. I always tried to spend time and speak with all of my patients. Just as a way to say that I was no different from them and that I was not conceited, as some people unfortunately become as doctors. I always thought it was very important to remember your roots and where you came from. I noticed that the patient's mom had been in the Emergency Room for quite a while, so I asked her whether she was hungry. She replied "Yes", so I offered to walk her to the cafeteria. I was not only being nice by doing this, but what she didn't know was that I had a trick up my sleeve.

During the entire trip to the cafeteria, I drilled her with questions about her son's disease. I wanted to learn more about it firsthand. I found out that her son was the only child affected with SCA in her family. She told me that during changes in weather, he tends to sickle, and he has to stay hydrated to avoid a sickling crisis. I also found out that he takes a medication called Hydroxyurea, which converts adult hemoglobin into fetal hemoglobin. This subsequently increases the oxygen level in his blood. I learned a lot more in that short three-hour shadowing session than weeks in the classroom, and couldn't wait to do it again.

Second year of medical school was more interesting and clinically applicable, but was also more challenging. We took classes such as Pathology, Pharmacology, Microbiology, Immunology, and studied disciplines such as Cardiology, Psychiatry, Orthopedics, Pediatrics, Radiology, and Neurosurgery. We even had the opportunity to visit the coroners' office and assisted in an autopsy, which I thought was incredibly interesting.

My patient at the coroner's office was an African American male who had died from an apparent heart attack while at home. The report we received before starting the autopsy was that he had a heart attack a few years prior, bad kidney disease, diabetes, and high blood pressure. He was also a heavy alcohol drinker and cocaine user. I glanced over at my classmates and said, "Wow, he was a disaster waiting to blow." Apparently he was found unresponsive in his apartment, lying on his belly, by his nephew who called 911.

As we unwrapped his body, I was quickly taken aback. He was no more than 45 years old, and I couldn't help but stare at his limp and lifeless body on our autopsy table. All I could do was think about my friends who ran the streets with me over the years, and how this could have been any of us. He was another black male who had likely left behind kids and a family. He was now gone forever, likely from something preventable.

Before starting the autopsy, we took several photos to use for evidence later. We then washed his body down with soap and water to remove the excess blood. As we examined his upper body, we found multiple marks on each arm. These were likely from injecting himself with cocaine and other drugs over the years. In addition, there was a catheter in his right forearm, which he probably used for dialysis. We then unwrapped the lower portion of his body and noticed that he was missing one leg.

"He probably never took his medication and his high blood pressure and diabetes got out of hand which lead to an amputation," I stated to my classmate, who nodded and agreed with me.

We made a "Y-shaped" incision, using a 10mm surgical blade, to enter his thoracic cavity and headed straight for his heart. We then used a pair of shears to cut his ribs bilaterally and lifted his rib cage by pulling it anteriorly, exposing his chest wall. We made several incisions along both sides of his heart and removed it from his chest for weighing and inspection. His heart weighed 490 grams, heavier than a normal heart of 350 grams. The heart muscle remodels itself and undergoes what we call hypertrophy, due to the stress from uncontrolled high blood pressure – the cause of his enlarged heart. We continued with our examination and looked at the most important artery in the heart, the left anterior descending artery (LAD). This artery delivers oxygen and nutrients to the heart, and blockage of it leads to a heart attack. We noticed right away, after we cut it open, that it had extensive areas of yellow calcification. It was very hard to the touch, a condition called atherosclerosis. We attempted to glance down the diameter of the vessel, but found it difficult to do. It had to be more than 90% occluded, which explained why he had the heart attack. We examined his remaining heart vessels and found they were occluded as well. I shook my head in disbelief and thought to myself, *This gentleman died of a massive heart attack, at a very young age. This could have easily been prevented.*

Growing up, I often noticed how my friends never went to the doctor. Whether from not having insurance or because they were ashamed to go, I never knew why. No one talked about high blood pressure, diabetes, heart disease, or kidney disease and about how these deadly diseases are interconnected and dangerous. No one ever wanted to talk about it. Once they did, it was already too late.

ADVICE:

Hypertension (HTN), or high blood pressure affects African Americans in unique ways. First, African Americans develop high blood pressure at younger ages than other groups in the US. In addition, they are more likely to develop complications from it such as stroke, heart disease, blindness, dementia, and kidney disease. In the U.S., the two leading causes of kidney failure are diabetes and high blood pressure. When the kidneys stop functioning properly, one requires dialysis or a kidney transplant to sustain life.

Here is some information about HTN, also called "the silent killer."

What is hypertension?
- A common condition in which the pressure of the blood in your blood vessels is higher than it should be

How common is hypertension?
- Very! About one in three U.S. adults, or 67 million people have high blood pressure
- Only about half (47%) of these people have it under control
- Costs the nation $47.5 billion each year, which includes the costs of healthcare services, medications for treatment, and missed days of work

What are some symptoms of hypertension?
- HTN is known as the "silent killer" because it often has no warning signs and most people don't know that they have it

- There is only one way for you to know if you have it: have a doctor or other health professional measure it

What do the blood pressure numbers mean?
- Blood pressure is measured using two numbers. The first number, called **systolic** blood pressure, represents the pressure in your blood vessels when your heart beats
- The second number, called **diastolic** blood pressure, represents the pressure in your blood vessels when your heart rests between beats
- A blood pressure of 120/80 is considered normal for most people
- If the number gets higher than this, your provider may want to modify your diet or start you on blood pressure medications

What are some unhealthy behaviors that can cause high blood pressure?
- Smoking tobacco
- Eating foods high in sodium and low in potassium
- Being overweight
- Drinking too much alcohol
- Not exercising enough

What can you do to lower or prevent high blood pressure?
- A lot of African Americans tend to have high blood pressure because it runs in their family (hereditary), but here are some things you can do to prevent it from getting too high:
  - Losing even ten pounds can lower your blood pressure. Losing weight has the biggest effect on those who are overweight and already have high blood pressure

o Eat healthy foods low in saturated fats, trans fat and cholesterol

o Minimize using salt. A half teaspoon of salt can raise your blood pressure as much as five millimeters of mercury

o Eat a diet that emphasizes fruits, vegetables and low-fat dairy products

o Increase your physical activity

o Limit alcohol to no more than one drink a day for women and no more than two drinks for men

o Stop smoking

...

At the end of second year of medical school, medical boards are taken. The exam is called the United States Medical Licensing Exam (USMLE), and is administered by the National Board of Medical Examiners. It is broken down into four separate exams. The first part of the exam, called Step One, is an eight-hour exam that essentially tests knowledge of the entire first and second year of medical school. After passing the brutal exam, we were able to progress to our clinical years of medical school. Most medical schools give you time to prepare for the exam. Knowing that I historically wasn't the best test taker, I made it a point to do as many practice questions as possible. I studied for six weeks straight and did almost 5,000 practice questions before sitting for the exam.

Our last requirement before heading into the hospital, during third year of medical school, involved a full day of orientation. This entailed receiving lectures from the Dean of the medical school, Clerkship directors, and hospital personnel. The Vice President of Georgetown Hospital then presented us with a riveting lecture about a medical student who had made a mistake and killed a patient. Apparently, a resident physician some years ago told a medical student to remove a central line (an IV catheter used to monitor patient's fluid status and also used to infuse large amounts of medications, fluids, etc.) from a patient. When the medical student went to remove the line, he didn't take the necessary steps to prevent air from getting into the patient's IV line. When he pulled the line out, the patient took a breath and breathed air into his IV line. The patient died within 30 seconds. This resonated within each and every one of my classmates and myself. It made us realize that any mistake made in the hospital, as simple as removing an IV line from a patient, could be detrimental and cost a patient his or her life.

Our third and fourth years of medical school were spent in the hospital, where we saw patients and essentially learned medicine hands on. Most people seemed to enjoy these years. This was because we were not forced to sit in a classroom all day. Instead, we actually went to work each day. There was a lottery process that allowed us to enter our preferences about which order we wanted to do our hospital rotations. Some people choose to do Surgery first and others choose to ease into third year by doing a lighter, less stressful rotation, such as Family Medicine. It was a somewhat strategic process and the order of your rotations dictated how your year went.

Starting clinical rotations in the hospital marked an exciting time in my career. I was finally able to begin living my lifelong dream of working in the hospital and taking care of patients. I was also one step closer to becoming a doctor. Being in the hospital, however, meant more responsibilities. Now, my actions were instrumental because patient's lives were in my hands and they depended on my medical expertise.

The majority of the time, I was the first person to see the patient early in the morning, usually around 5:30 am. On my Surgery rotation, it was sometimes as early as 4:15 am. We, as medical students, were then responsible for reporting and presenting during rounds to the head doctor, whom we called the "Attending." Rounds was when a team of individuals, ranging from nurses, doctors, respiratory therapists, pharmacists and students, got together and discussed the symptoms of each patient. We then came up with ideas about what could have been causing the patient's symptoms and came up with differentials (list of possible diagnoses). This was followed by "pimping." Pimping was when the head doctors drilled us with back-to-back questions.

"What is the association between polycystic kidney disease and this patient's headache?"

"What are the side effects of furosemide that you need to worry about once we give it to our patient?"

"What is the latest consensus on using rate control versus rhythm control in our patient with atrial fibrillation?"

Back to back, non-stop questions, tested how much we studied the night before and how we reacted under pressure. This entailed not only knowing our physical exam findings, but also having some knowledge of the patient's disease process and pathogenesis. This was a time to shine if you knew your information or a time of embarrassment, in front of all your superiors and colleagues, if you were asked a question and didn't know the answer.

During this year, the majority of students also chose their specialty of choice. In medicine, depending on your grades, clerkship evaluations, and letters of recommendation, there are several possibilities when deciding on a specialty. For the months leading up to this, I prayed and asked God for guidance. I also spoke with mentors and friends about which direction I should take in my medical career. As a first year medical student, one of my professors broke it down succinctly. He stated, "When making a career decision, one should think about four things: Money, prestige, lifestyle and passion." For example, if one chooses to become a Neurosurgeon, which is an extremely competitive field to enter into, he or she will have the prestige and respect of almost every physician and make tons of money ($500k to over 1 million a year), but sacrifice family time and neglect lifestyle. He or she will make lots of money, but will be working so much that he/she will not be able to enjoy it. He will most likely miss those baseball and basketball games for his son and most likely miss nightly dinner times with his family. Conversely, one who decides to go into Pediatrics will sacrifice compensation (they are some of the lowest paid physicians averaging around $125k-$150k a year) for lifestyle (you will have more time off) and prestige (not very prestigious). As I planned my last year of medical school and prayed about which specialty to practice medicine in, I took in account all of those factors. For me, lifestyle played the largest part in my decision making process. Compensation, a little less so. Choosing a specialty based on how much money you will make was highly discouraged by our predecessors. Changes in the US healthcare system, which will take place over the next 5-10 years, will dramatically change how much physicians are paid. Medicare payments to physicians are predicted to be cut by nearly 30%. That same physician who made $400k five years ago may easily see a $100k pay cut. So, basing your decision on how much you will get paid was not advised.

A Chinese philosopher and teacher, named Confucius, once said, "Choose a job you love and you will never have to work a day in your life." These words made me realize that you really have to pick a specialty which you have a passion for. I always knew that I worked well in chaotic environments. I also loved working with my hands, like doing procedures and surgeries. I vividly remembered those years working in the ICU when I got an adrenaline rush as patients came in very sick and on the verge of death with gunshot wounds and mangled extremities. Those critical minutes and decision-making moments meant whatever decision we made, would make the difference between life and death for that patient. Most would argue that being in a situation like that for years on end can eventually lead to physician burnout and unneeded stress, something that I also had to consider when I made my decision.

At the end of medical school, in our fourth year, we applied to postgraduate training, also known as residency. Applying to residency was just as competitive or somewhat more competitive than applying to medical school. I spent a good portion of this year traveling to different cities, visiting hospitals, and searching for potential employers. Interviews, especially for surgery, were quite intimidating and completely random.

When I interviewed at Harvard University, I was told to give my best Boston accent. That was my first time in Boston, but luckily I overheard someone yelling at someone else the night before. I essentially repeated what I heard. When I walked into the interview room while at Wake Forest, I was told "Don't sit down. Go back outside! You have five minutes to come up with something non-medical to teach us using the white board." I gave the surgeons a confused look and nervously walked back out of the room. I went back into the room three minutes later and taught them about military customs and courtesies. In the middle of my interview at Stanford, the surgeon took out a blank piece of paper and said, "I want you to draw me the proximal femur with all the muscle origins, insertions, blood and nerve supply." I knew I wasn't the best drawer, so I had to improvise. I tried my best and drew a femur showing the attachment of the external rotators to the greater trochanter. He essentially wanted to see how I reacted under pressure, a trait essential in surgery.

After interviews, we ranked the programs where we interviewed. We placed our top programs higher on the list, and the programs we did not like at the bottom of our lists. The interviewing programs did the same for each applicant that they interviewed. A very complex algorithm was then applied to generate a match list, which informed medical students whether they "matched" or not. Every medical school around the country has a Match Day in March of each year. This was when we found out if and where we matched for residency. This was a very exciting time for some and very upsetting time for others. Most people matched at their top choice of residency location, but unfortunately some did not match at all. When this happens, you are forced to take whatever job is open at that time.

Each residency program, depending on the specialty, has between three to eight spots. Some programs have more spots and some have less. Some of the more competitive residency fields included: Neurosurgery, Plastic Surgery, Orthopedic Surgery, Dermatology and Urology. These specialty fields were the hardest to match into and required high medical board examination scores, good grades and well-written letters of recommendations from respectable faculty members.

I always knew that I wanted to be a surgeon, primarily because I loved working with my hands. Surgery is competitive, intense, fast paced and life changing. The ability to make a intervention that produces immediate results fascinated me the most. Knowing that Orthopedic Surgery was one of the most competitive fields to enter into, I studied hard and spent endless hours studying for exams, to ensure I made the best grades obtainable. I often spent 16-20 hours a day studying in the library and then slept for two to three hours. I woke up in the morning and repeated that process again. This meant I sacrificed going out with classmates, spending time with friends and family, and personal time. Having to compete with my medical school classmates, who were from various Ivy League schools such as Harvard, Yale, and Princeton, on exams was a challenge in itself. I will admit, I am not the brightest person in the world, but if you put me in a room with a pack of wolves, I will come out victorious.

Thomas Edison once said, "Genius is one percent inspiration and ninety-nine percent perspiration." If my classmates, from those Ivy League schools, read a chapter on a subject once, I read that same chapter three times, reinforcing the knowledge over and over. Essentially, it meant working harder than the person who was next to me.

You will find in life that many of your colleagues and associates are some of the brightest and most intelligent people you have ever met. Don't let this discourage you from reaching your dreams and achieving your full potential. Come to work 30 minutes early, go home and review that topic no one knew about during the employee meeting, or stay 20 minutes later than everyone else. It will pay off in the end.

Vince Lombardi once said, "The dictionary is the only place that success comes before work. Work is the key to success, and hard work can help you accomplish anything." I accomplished exactly what I wanted, which was to become an Orthopedic Surgeon. Mainly, because I sacrificed so much during my childhood years, time in the military and while at Georgetown. It finally paid off. Not only did I match into the field of Orthopedic Surgery, but I also was invited to interview at some of those Ivy League schools that my classmates once attended for undergraduate studies. These were places I had always dreamt of attending while applying to medical school. I interviewed at Harvard University, Cleveland Clinic, Baylor University, Wake Forest, SUNY Upstate, Northwestern University, Ohio State University, Tulane University, and Stanford University to name a few. My hard work and countless hours of studying finally had paid off. It was a 360-degree turn from applying to medical school, after essentially praying and hoping for interview invites. Instead, I found myself with 15 + residency job offers, in one of the most competitive specialties in medicine.

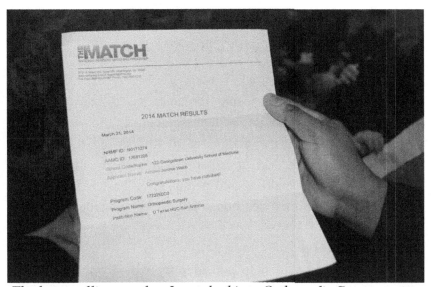

The letter telling me that I matched into Orthopedic Surgery at my # 1 spot

ADVICE:

The first step in choosing a career is to know yourself. Whether you are a first year college student, a third year medical student preparing for the match, or a 40-year-old teacher with hopes of changing careers, it is paramount that you first identify your interests, values, skills, and personality. This will allow you to make a well-informed decision when deciding on a career.

Your Interests

Your interests will help you identify which opportunities to pursue, and know which topics you are most naturally drawn towards. This will make the schooling process and work afterwards more enjoyable. Are you interested in science or biology? If not, then medicine may not be for you. Are you interested in math or good with numbers? Then, maybe finance or account management will be a good career field for you. Are you investigative and like to analyze or interpret ambiguous data? Maybe forensic science or homicide investigator is the field for you.

Your Values

Your values are the things that help you move towards certain decisions, behaviors, and goals, and motivate you to keep going. Your values are what will influence your career decision, the decision-making process, job satisfaction, and – ultimately – life satisfaction. Visit www.lifevaluesinventory.org for a free online value quiz that was developed to help people, like yourself, clarify values and serve as a blueprint for effective career decision making.

Your Skills

Your skills are things that you are good at and have the ability to do well. Assessing your skills will give you an indication of what field you may be good at. Growing up, I was always good at building things and loved working with my hands. I was immediately drawn to surgery the moment I first stepped foot in the operating room. If you find that you enjoy and are good at talking in front of groups of people, maybe teaching will be right for you.

Your Personality

Your personality is related to your individual, innate nature and tends not to change over time. Understanding this will allow you to see correlations between the way you make decisions and your work style. Surgeons are thought to be abrasive, extroverts, arrogant, hostile and cantankerous at times. I'm not saying all surgeons possess these personality traits, but if these are not characteristics that describe you, then surgery may not be for you. Teachers tend to be compassionate, patient, creative and optimistic. If this sounds like it paints a picture of you, then you may want to consider teaching.

There are many traps and wrong ways to go about choosing a career. Here are tips to avoid them:

Picking a career based on pay

Choosing a career based on its schedule or how much money you will make means you are choosing a job, rather than a career. You may make decent money for a few years, but will you still be happy and eager to go to work each day years down the line? You want to choose a career where even when you have to get up at 4:00 am and head to work, you will still enjoy doing it years later. I would hate for someone to go through 10-15 years of training to become a doctor, just for the money, and have no passion for helping others. Make a list of the pros and cons of your potential career field. If the cons outweigh the pros, then that career may not be for you.

Picking a career because everyone says you will be good at it

I saw this many times in medical school. The majority of my classmates had parents and family members who were doctors. Growing up, their family constantly pushed the idea of medicine as a career and enrolled them in prep courses, medical academies and preparatory schools. Once they actually got into medical school, they hated it. Don't fall for this trap. Don't pick a career because everyone is doing it or just because your parents tell you to choose it. You will be the one who will be getting up each morning and going to your job ten years down the line. So, make it your decision and make sure to pick something you enjoy doing.

Picking a career that will cost you more money to fund your education than you will ever make

I once met an individual by the name of Sam. Sam was a very intelligent person and was streetwise, but not very book smart. He told me he was finishing up school at a local university and would be graduating soon. I asked him what he was going to do with his degree afterwards and his response baffled me.

"I don't know, I haven't thought that far out yet," he responded.

He just spent four years of his life on school and racked up $160,000 in student loans. Don't fall for this trap. When you are choosing a career and decide on a school to attend, make sure you consider your return on investment (ROI). Essentially, this is your investment gains as compared to your investment costs. When it comes to ROI and education, not all degrees are considered equal.

To calculate ROI for a specific degree, first determine the overall cost of the degree. Know that this amount will be higher if you attend a private institution versus a public school. Make sure you include all books and fees including room and board. Next, obtain the median cash compensation over the course of the next 30 years. You can obtain this information from salary.com, but be sure to include inflation and cost of living. Finally, subtract the cost of the degree from gains over 30 years and divide that by cost.

Salary.com listed eight college degrees that have the worst return on investment. People who enter the field of Sociology and enter careers as Social Workers have low or negative ROIs. Corrections officers or Counselors also tend not to have very positive ROIs.

For example, the median salary of a social worker is $47,121 per year with 30-year earnings of $2,779,195. After attending a public university for four years to obtain this degree, your ROI would be 73% and 21% if you attended a private college. Conversely, if you have good problem solving skills and a gift for developing products, devices and systems, a degree in engineering will earn you your money back. According to salary.com, the median salary of an Electrical Engineering Supervisor is $91,997 with 30-year earnings of $5,425,980. Attending a public university for four years will give you a ROI of 144% and private university will give you 44%.

Education is an investment, so invest wisely!

NEVER JUDGE A BOOK BY ITS COVER

Are you a basketball player? You *must* play sports."
I didn't even get the chance to sit down in my seat, when an older white lady on my flight back to DC started bombarding me with questions. I politely informed her that I was actually studying to become a doctor. Immediately, her eyes grew *big*! After that, her whole demeanor changed and we had a great conversation the rest of the flight back to DC.

The year prior, during a Thanksgiving holiday break from medical school, I decided to travel to New York to visit family members who were stationed at the US Military Academy at West Point. I gathered my bags and left for the bus stop, eagerly looking forward to a nice break filled with stuffed turkey, dressing, and my favorite, pecan pie. In medical school, every chance you get to study, you study. Whether reading notes in line at the grocery store, reviewing flashcards while out eating with friends, or listening to a recorded lecture audio at the gym, every opportunity to study is taken advantage of.

Once I arrived in New York and got off the bus, I called my aunt and waited for her to come pick me up. While waiting, I decided to pull out my Anatomy book and review for an upcoming exam. We had just taken our physiology portion of the exam for Cardiopulmonary and would be tested on the anatomy part after the holiday break. I pulled out my anatomy book, put my headphones on, and started studying. Minutes later, I felt a tap on my shoulder. I looked up to see who it was. *Maybe it was someone who recognized me or maybe someone I went to school with back in the day, and was just saying hello*, I thought. But wait, I was in

New York. It was very unlikely that someone would know me there. Still, I was surprised when I looked up and saw an older white male, in a police officer uniform. He stated that he wanted to speak with me.

Startled, I asked him, "Excuse me, is there a problem sir?"

He responded with a strong New York accent, "I need to speak with you. You fit the description of a male who we are looking for that just stole something from one of the mall stores."

I couldn't believe what I just heard. There I was, sitting down and minding my own business, studying an anatomy book of all things, and I was approached because I looked *"suspicious?"* Everyone else, waiting at the bus, stopped and looked in our direction trying to see what the commotion was about. I had heard many stories of black males resisting arrest or not being cooperative with officers, and getting shot or killed as a result. I definitely wanted to avoid that from happening.

"I am studying. I have no clue what you are talking about. I would appreciate it if you would just leave."

I kept my voice stern and demanding. He apparently heard the frustration in my voice and turned around and walked away.

It happened again, years later, while I was working out at the gym. Out of nowhere, an older gentleman approached me and started talking. I couldn't hear what he was saying, because I had my earphones in. After stopping my music, he said, "You look like a salesman."

I gave him a very confused look and said, "What makes you think that? I'm actually a doctor."

Was it maybe something that I was wearing? The way I was carrying myself? Or, maybe because I was one of the only black males working out in the gym that day? Who knows?

He immediately said, "Oh I'm sorry, I'm very proud of you" and extended his hand for a handshake.

For the rest of my workout, I couldn't help but ask myself why he thought I was a salesman, just by looking at me.

While working in the ICU at Wilford Hall Medical Center in 2008, I met a gentleman by the name of Juan. Juan was a quiet, reserved, and laid back fellow who had served time in the military and gotten out on military disability. To make time go by faster and to make a little extra change, he got a job at the ICU. He worked as one of our administrators – essentially a secretary who filed our paperwork, shredded papers, etc. Everyone thought Juan was a little weird. He didn't say much. He just came to work, did his job, and went home.

One day, I decided to start a conversation with him. At the time, I was really interested in real estate. I wanted to start my own business of buying and selling real estate in Texas. And, San Antonio was the prime market for it. I even moved one of my best friends from Shreveport to San Antonio to start up and run the company. After talking to Juan one day, I learned that he had been buying and selling houses for years, making hundreds of thousands of dollars in profit. We had a long conversation about the process of searching for properties, how to buy them, and how to find good deals. He even gave me some of his contacts. At the end of our conversation, he wanted to show me something on the computer. He logged into his account and what popped up took me by surprise. He had $550,000 in his investment account! The guy who everyone treated like "a nobody" and who was "just our secretary" had over a half million dollars in his investment account. He had another $450,000 in other accounts.

"The doctors here talk to me and treat me like crap," he said, with a shake of his head. "Like I'm a nobody. Promise me you'll never judge people by how they look or act when you become a doctor."

He logged off the computer and walked away, leaving me speechless and with a new motto to live by: Never judge a book by its cover.

ADVICE:

We live in a very superficial society where people have preconceived notions based on what they see on the surface, without taking the time to delve deeper. In Samuel 16:7, the Bible says, "The Lord does not look at the things man looks at. Man looks at the outward appearance, but the Lord looks at the heart." A person's appearance, physical attributes, or how they dress may not be any indication of their inner well-being. Humans are incredibly complex individuals. While their physical appearance may well be apparent, their spiritual (inner) dimension is not. So, remember this the next time your intuition tells you to form an assumption about a person based on how they look or act. You never know who that person may be, or how they could be a blessing to your life.

THE UNEXPECTED

I always knew something was a little different. Something just didn't seem right. I repressed thoughts of it, until I had to face it. The realization came, one gloomy day, during my 2nd year of medical school.

"Which medications are you taking, Mom?" I paused while she answered. "What are you taking those for?"

In medical school, we learned hundreds of different types of drugs, their side effects, and clinical use. I became very familiar with the most commonly used medications for Cardiac, Neurological, Respiratory, and Psychiatric diseases. I was shocked to find out, and never imagined, that my mother and sister would be taking several medications that we had recently learned about in Psychiatry.

I was 28 years old, and a second year medical student when I first learned that my mom and sister both have schizophrenia. I was in denial at first, but then it began to all make sense. Schizophrenia explained the numerous hospitalizations, ER visits, and run-ins with the police that occurred over the years. Similar to my mom, my little sister first started hearing voices when she was just 14 years old.

"Mom, I see someone over there. They're trying to get me."

My sister and mom were on the city bus and headed to the grocery store, when my sister started hallucinating. She explained to my mom that she saw imaginary people and they were trying to harm her.

"There is no one over there. You're just seeing things," my mom told her. She tried to calm my sister down. They then went on with their day and my mom did not think anything else of it.

But the hallucinations came back.

Weeks later, my sister was at home when she heard more voices. The voices told her to hurt herself. When my dad found out, he immediately took her to the Emergency Room. From the ER, she was sent to a mental hospital in Shreveport, called Brentwood. After some testing, she was diagnosed with Schizophrenia. I wouldn't learn about this diagnosis until my second year in medical school. Growing up, I knew she was always in and out of the hospital, but I never knew why. At Brentwood, she was placed on psychiatric medications, though the hallucinations and voices never fully stopped. Even while undergoing treatment, she continued to hear voices. One voice told her to hang herself. Another voice told her to slash her wrist.

She listened to those voices.

She tried to slash her wrist and then attempted to hang herself. The psychiatrist, who was on duty that day, called my father and informed him what had happened. My father broke down in tears. He was puzzled and demanded an answer. His daughter had been normal for 14 years before that. Now, she was in the hospital and had just tried to commit suicide. He didn't understand why.

The psychiatrist adjusted her medications and the voices soon went away. She spent several weeks hospitalized on the psychiatric ward before she was discharged home.

Nicole was just a young kid when she began her battle with Schizophrenia. She was constantly challenged, on a daily basis, with the task of whether to listen to the voices in her head or to listen to what was really happening in reality. No young kid wants to take medication on a daily basis. No kid wants to sit in a hospital room, for weeks at a time, while doctors try to find the perfect balance of medication for your condition. Young kids like to feel cool and accepted. They often go out of their way to do so. There was nothing cool about taking medication. Nothing cool about constantly going to the mental hospital. This may have been what led Nicole to stop taking her medications. It was also when things started going downhill.

People with Schizophrenia may hear voices that other people don't. Sometimes the voices may tell them to harm themselves. Schizophrenia may also lead people to have false beliefs, such as the belief that they are God or have supernatural powers. Such beliefs often lead to altercations and disputes with the police. The majority of the time, this occurs when people use drugs or stop taking their medications concomitantly with their Schizophrenia. That was exactly what happened to my sister. She stopped taking her medication and ended up in prison on two felony charges.

Many days, during her time in prison, she was placed on 23-hour lockdown. During those times, she was forced to sit in her jail cell for 23 hours straight. She was only allowed to be out of her cell for one hour, to shower and get fresh air. Her food was handed to her through a small opening in the prison bars, called a "food hatch." While on lockdown, she slept on the hard, concrete floor without a pillow or blanket. During that time, the hallucinations returned. This eventually lead to verbal altercations between the prison officers and my sister. The officers were unaware of her mental illness and need for medication. Instead, she was sentenced to more days on lockdown. It was not until my father called the prison, that she was transferred to the psychiatric ward where her medications were restarted.

When medications are stopped, patients with Schizophrenia become psychotic again. This leads to repeat hospital visits and creates a great deal of turmoil for the patient and their family. Non-adherence with medications can become a problem, especially if there is a concurrent substance abuse. Drugs such as marijuana and cocaine can lead to relapse and make symptoms worse.

Schizophrenia often goes undiagnosed for many years. Before the diagnosis is made, altercations with the police, domestic disputes, and other criminal activities usually occur. The diagnosis often manifests itself at vital life stages, interrupting education and training. This places those affected at a disadvantage in the labor market. While Schizophrenia is not a very common disorder, it is one of the most disabling mental disorders, and the most misunderstood.

ADVICE:

What is Schizophrenia?
- A chronic, severe brain disorder that affects how a person thinks, feels and acts
- Comes from the Greek word *skhizein* meaning "to split" and the Greek word *Phrenos* meaning "diaphragm, heart, mind."
- People with Schizophrenia may have a hard time distinguishing between what is real and what is imaginary
- People with Schizophrenia may hear voices other people don't hear
- People with Schizophrenia may believe other people are reading their minds, controlling their thoughts, or plotting to harm them

What Schizophrenia is NOT
- A split or multiple personality
- A violent or dangerous condition to others
- Caused by childhood experiences or poor parenting

What causes Schizophrenia?
- The exact cause is unclear
- Theories include: genetics (hereditary), biology (the imbalance in the chemistry of the brain) and/or possible viral infections and autoimmune disorders

How common is Schizophrenia?
- Affects approximately 1.4 million people or about 1% of Americans

- 40 percent of the homeless roaming the streets have Schizophrenia

What are some early warning signs?
- Hearing or seeing things that aren't there
- Inappropriate or bizarre behavior
- A change in personal hygiene and appearance
- A constant feeling of being watched
- Increasing withdrawal from social situations
- Inability to sleep or concentrate

What treatments are available?
- If you suspect you or someone you know is experiencing symptoms of Schizophrenia, encourage them to see a medical or mental health professional immediately
- Because the causes of Schizophrenia are still unknown, treatment focuses on eliminating the symptoms of the disease
- Medications, group therapy, social and vocational rehabilitation are some available treatment modalities
- Early treatment can mean a better long-term outcome

Resources
- National Alliance for the Mentally Ill (NAMI)
  1-800-950-NAM
  www.nami.org

- National Alliance for Research on Schizophrenia and Depression (NARSD)
  1-800-829-8289
  www.narsad.org

"I'M DONE"

I'M DONE!" Words you never want to hear from a trauma surgeon. It was 2:00 am in the Trauma Intensive Care unit, during my last rotation of medical school, when my pager began beeping loudly in tandem with an overhead message. A code blue – the code for a very sick person who required immediate assistance – was en route to the ER with an estimated time of arrival of ten minutes. The resident grabbed my arm as he hurried past me in the direction of the ER.

"Shall we do this?" he asked, voice dripping with sarcasm.

Knowing that whenever a code blue trauma came in, anything could happen, we prepared ourselves for the worst possible scenario. We rushed to the emergency room only to be met by 10-15 other people all dressed in PPA (personal protective attire). This meant shoe covers, long gowns, masks, head covers and gloves – all of which are worn to protect one from bodily fluids such as blood, saliva or vomit. Patients that enter the ER can carry any sort of disease imaginable – it would be all too easy to contract HIV or hepatitis from a patient, if splashed in the eye with blood or stuck by a needle. One could never be too careful.

I made a quick assessment to determine who was already in the trauma bay. There was an Anesthesiologist, an ICU nurse, the head trauma surgeon, General Surgery and Emergency Medicine residents, Respiratory therapists, a scribe, and medical students. Everyone in the room has an assigned role during the trauma, and stands at specific positions around the injured patient's bed. At the head of the bed is the Anesthesiologist and Respiratory therapist. They are responsible for maintaining a patent airway and utilization of an artificial breathing tube and machine, if needed. To the right of the patient stands the general surgery resident. This

153

person is responsible for quickly assessing the patient, from the moment he enters the trauma bay, for life-threating injuries and performing diagnostic or therapeutic procedures. Standing close by would be an ICU nurse, who listens in closely and observes. If the patient lived long enough to make it to the ICU, the ICU nurse will know exactly what happened to the patient, from the moment they hit the trauma door. At the back of the room stands the head trauma surgeon and scribe. Despite all the chaotic yelling, the scribe's job is to quickly jot down notes and capture key vital signs, medications given, and orders placed. The head trauma surgeon sits back and observes, barking out orders to everyone, to make sure everything runs smoothly.

After I donned my gear and found a pair of gloves, that awkward moment of silence kicked in — where everyone expected the unexpected to happen at any minute. In trauma, anything can happen at any minute. A stable patient can become unstable and make a turn for the worse at a moment's notice. The inevitable questions began to trickle into my mind. Would this patient make it? Would we be able to save him?

Moments later, the door to the front of the ER was kicked open and the first thing I saw was a big machine pounding on the patient's – an older gentleman's – chest. His heart had stopped beating en route to the hospital and required restarting with an automatic compression machine called a Lucas. This machine repeatedly applied compressions to his chest as they wheeled him toward our trauma bed. When I saw this, my own heart sank. We weren't off to a good start.

"We have a 50ish year old male," the paramedic yelled out. "Gunshot wound to his chest with an exit wound to his left flank. He went into PEA arrest en route, and we placed a endotracheal tube for airway support."

PEA is short for pulseless electrical activity – a heart rhythm that requires immediate pharmacological intervention. It would take everything we had to save this man – and then some.

"Do we have a blood pressure?" yelled the head trauma surgeon.

Suddenly, the ER was a flurry of activity – everyone working as hard and as fast as they could, doing everything possible to save the gentleman.

His blood pressure was low – so low, in fact, that we knew we didn't have much time. I quickly began cutting his clothes off with my trauma shears so I could further assess his injuries and potentially stop any visible bleeding. But, I didn't see any. He continued to crash fast. We gave him multiple liters of blood and fluid. Despite that, we still could not get his blood pressure to rise.

It was time to make a quick decision.

Because of the gunshot wound, it was likely that fluid had surrounded his heart and was now compressing it. We had no choice but to open his chest and relieve the pressure.

"Give me the thoracotomy tray, we need to open him up," yelled the general surgery chief resident.

Even though I was near completion of medical school and had even served in war as a combat medic, I had only seen this procedure done once. I also knew that patients who require this life-saving procedure almost never made it out of the hospital.

Within seconds, the chief resident surgeon had taken a scalpel and made a large incision over this gentleman's chest, right over his heart. Then, an echoing, blood-chilling *snap* echoed the room as he used large retractors to break the patient's ribs. Now, he could fully access his heart.

Blood spurted in every direction and covered the ER floor, including our clean scrubs and white shoes.

Once inside the heart cavity, the resident massaged the patient's heart with his hands, which would hopefully restore blood flow. Even if this gentleman lived, he would have suffered massive neurological damage from blood loss to his brain. The situation looked bleak.

While the nurses helped place additional IVs for more fluids, and the respiratory therapist poked the man's scrawny arm to draw blood, the chief resident continued massaging his heart, now with even more force.

"His heart is becoming dry, we need more fluids," he yelled.

He then looked down and noticed something that made him gasp – a tiny hole in the man's lung that appeared to be oozing blood.

"We have a leakage," he screamed.

The gunshot had not only pierced his chest, but had hit his lung as well, causing massive bleeding inside the chest cavity. I realized that was likely the reason we couldn't get his blood pressure up. Regardless, if we couldn't stop the bleeding, he wouldn't survive much longer.

"Pack him up!" screamed the head trauma surgeon. "We're going to the operating room."

At this time, I was awed by what I had just witnessed. I was told that the best way to get involved as a medical student, was to just jump in and help. I immediately started grabbing things that we would need en route to the operating room and placed them on the bed. Within seconds, we were rushing out of the ER and heading to the operating room. Blood was everywhere and trails of it were left behind as we quickly ran and pushed this gentleman's bed in the direction of the OR 6.

We overheard that his family was outside the trauma bay, waiting anxiously, but our main focus was saving this man's life. As we wheeled the bed out of the trauma bay, I noticed a distraught family in the corner of my eye. I could not muster up the courage to make eye contact with them, as I knew in my heart that things were not going well. In all honesty, what we were doing was probably futile at that point.

We sped towards the operating room, screaming at people who were up ahead, to move out of our path. Adrenaline raced through my veins as I drew in a panicked breath.

It was when we made it to the operating room, and were in the process of transferring him to the OR bed from the trauma stretcher, that the respiratory therapist noticed his heart was beating on its own.

I glanced over to look inside his chest and, indeed, his heart was beating. But, it didn't stay that way for long. Once again, his heart rate slowly dwindled away and the resident surgeon was forced to continue massaging his heart.

"We need to stop the bleeding from his lung, otherwise he would exsanguinate right before our eyes," I mumbled to myself.

We quickly performed a procedure where we used a scalpel to cut a portion of his lung out, and twisted it around itself forming a knot. The idea behind this was that the twisted portion of the lung may potentially stop and control the bleeding. It worked, but we all knew it was only a temporary fix.

His blood pressure now had dropped to 80/40.

Suddenly, a thought struck me. Knowing that I may never get the opportunity to perform a cardiac massage, I glanced over at the resident massaging the heart and asked, "Hey, do you think I can give this a try?"

He hesitated for a second, but then leaned over and ran it by the head trauma surgeon.

"Yes, but only for 10 seconds," he then stated.

I eagerly placed my right hand inside the patient's chest and grabbed his heart, which fitted perfectly in my hand. I squeezed his heart with all my might, and tried to squeeze it at a coordinated pace of one squeeze every few seconds. I realized, in that moment, that his life was literally in my hands. If I stopped squeezing his heart, he would die. I squeezed for about 45 seconds and then the trauma surgeon brushed me aside so he could take over again.

He got everyone's attention in the OR and said the words that no one ever wants to hear. "If his heart doesn't return after this next unit of blood, I'm done."

We had done everything we could do to save this patient's life, and spent thousands of dollars for a condition that has a very high mortality rate. Nonetheless, we kept resuscitating him with hopes of bringing him back. *Because that's what doctors do.* But, that never happened.

Several minutes later, we pronounced him dead.

In that moment, time seemed to stop. There was no more running around, no more cardiac massage, no more nurses rapidly infusing large amounts of fluids, and no more screams from the head surgeon. Everything stopped, just like that.

Slowly, the details began to trickle in. From what we gathered, the patient was an IV drug user, who tried to commit suicide by shooting himself in his chest. Apparently, he attempted suicide several times before but this time he succeeded.

ADVICE:

According to the Centers for Disease Control and Prevention, more people die of suicide than car accidents. In 2010, there were 33,687 deaths from motor vehicle crashes and 38,364 suicides. From 1999 to 2010, the suicide rate among Americans aged 35-64 rose by nearly 30% from 13.7 to 17.6 per 100,000 people. The majority of these suicides came from men in their 50s. In 2010, firearms were the most common method for completing suicide followed by suffocation (includes hangings) and poisoning.

If a friend or family member tells you that he or she is thinking about death or suicide, it's important to evaluate the immediate danger the person is in. Those at the highest risk for committing suicide have a specific suicide PLAN, the MEANS to carry out the plan, a SET TIME for doing it, and an INTENT to do it.

The following questions can help you assess the immediate risk for suicide:

Do you have a suicide plan? (PLAN)

Do you have what you need to carry out your plan (pills, gun, etc.)? (MEANS)

Do you know when you would do it? (SET TIME)

Do you intend to commit suicide? (INTENT)

If a suicide attempt seems imminent, call a local crisis center, 911, or take the person to an emergency room. Remove guns, drugs, knives, and other potentially lethal weapons from the vicinity. Do NOT, under any circumstance, leave a suicidal person alone.

THE HOPEFUL CHANGE

After seeing my little brother lay helpless in his hospital bed back in 2008, I promised myself as a medical student that I would empathize and show compassion to my own patients. Instead of just going through the day-to-day routine of my job, I made it a goal to spend more time with each patient on a daily basis. Clinicians are often caught up in the day-to-day business of being a physician. Unfortunately, simple assurances, once vowed to during the Hippocratic Oath as medical students, become neglected as a result.

Every medical school requires students to take the Hippocratic Oath, in one form or another, during medical school and at graduation. We vowed to respect and abide by principles such as beneficence, non-maleficence, patient autonomy, and social justice. We began our journey in medical school as ambitious, self-starting, compassionate, and empathetic learners of medicine. Our goal was to save the world, not knowing what real world medicine was really like. Not everyone loses this drive and passion. However, at some point during medical training the paradigm shifts. It changes from treating patients as Mr./Mrs. Jones to treating patient number 48 of 120 that you have to see that day.

A study published in the *Journal of General Internal Medicine* in 2007 showed that medical students lose empathy as they progress through their medical training. Six hundred fifty-eight students participated in the study and were administered the Jefferson Scale of Physician Empathy Questionnaire. First year medical students had the highest empathy scores, while fourth-year medical students had the lowest.

While empathy decreases over the years, the number of hours physicians are required to work increases. In addition, the time

161

provided to get all the work accomplished during the day decreases dramatically. During intern year of residency, one can expect to work 80-100 hours a week. Recently, the governing body of residency programs in the US mandated that residents and interns work a maximum number of hours each week. This was implemented primarily for safety concerns. Currently, that maximum amount is set at 80 hours a week. Most interns and residents will tell you that they commonly work more than 80 hours. They keep quiet due to the fear of being ostracized by fellow peers or being labeled as "the one who is complaining again." Most just suck it up and get the work done, even if it means sacrificing family or personal time. Patients have to be seen, procedures have to be carried out, prescriptions need to be filled, and discharges need to take place. All of which occurs while working scrupulously to not anger superiors, by working too slow or not doing something their specific way. Interns and residents alike were often left to provide care for 20-30 patients at a time, all individually requiring some type of special medical need.

During *my* intern year of residency, I was astounded to discover how much responsibility I had accrued as compared to my last year of medical school, which ended just several weeks prior. During medical school, we worked under the supervision of an upper level resident and attending physician. During that time, we only directly took care of one to four patients at maximum. Months later, during my first year as a doctor, that patient load suddenly increased to an average of 20-30 patients. I was the doctor responsible for ensuring no one died under my care.

We learned *thousands* of things in medical school over a four-year period. Similar to throwing mud on a wall, we were expected to take in monstrous amounts of information and regurgitate it at the bedside to take care of patients. The thought was this: If we saw the same medical condition repetitively, and reinforced it with lots of reading, eventually the mud would stick.

That knowledge would become vital during my first week of internship. I had been a doctor for less than a week when my pager went off informing me that my patient – who had undergone a major pelvic and shoulder surgery – wouldn't wake up or respond.

" Dr. Webb!! Your patient isn't responsive. Hurry!"

A few hours earlier that same nurse, Sally, had paged me because her other patient was breathing irregularly and his heart rate was high. I quickly ran through a list of potential deadly conditions in my head that could kill my patient, Mark, and tried to eliminate them. In medicine, we are trained to think that way, in order to provide immediate action, if needed. Could this be an aortic dissection? Myocardial infarction? Pulmonary embolism? I quickly ordered the nurse to get an EKG for his heart, a chest X-ray for his lungs, and ordered pain medicine (on the off chance that it could all be due to pain).

My pager went off again. It was a nurse upstairs on the 8th floor who wanted to discharge her patient. I glanced at Mark. He was still writhing and moaning in bed. His oxygen saturation began to slowly dwindle down. A learned trait during medical school and residency is prioritization. Essentially, this meant placing emphasis and attention on the most critically ill patient. Several nurses might page at once, which requires one to make the decision of which patient to see first.

I ignored the page from the nurse upstairs.

"Mark! Mark! Open your eyes," I yelled.

No response.

He was foaming from his mouth at that point, and his eyes had rolled back into his head. I rubbed my knuckles hard on his chest to see if he would respond.

"Mark, open your eyes!!"

By that point, several nurses and other intern colleagues arrived to see what all the commotion was about. I suddenly recalled my 2nd year of medical school pharmacology where I learned about a drug called Narcan. It's a drug used to reverse overdosed narcotic pain medicine.

"Give him 0.4mg of Narcan," I tried to shout authoritatively, but it came out mumbled and with uncertainty. Seconds later – though it seemed like hours – passed by and then Mark suddenly opened his eyes. He moaned and shouted out random words and phrases as if he was intoxicated. But, even though his words didn't make sense and he was confused, I was relieved that he was alive. I sure didn't want to be the intern who killed a patient his first week on the job.

I looked over at Sally, and she had a terrified look on her face.

"The strong narcotics must have sedated him too deeply," I told her. "What do you think we should do now?"

She looked me in my eyes and said, "I'm not sure. *You're* the doctor," and walked away.

Instances like that occurred all too often during my intern year, requiring me to make key medical decisions every day on the spot. Instead of taking the time to speak with my patients each morning, as I did while a medical student, I now found myself thinking of what I could do or say as an exit strategy before entering each room to see my 20+ patients. When I only had 45 minutes to see 17 patients, time became critical. I pray that I re-experience that same ambition and compassion that I encountered while seeing my little brother lay helpless in the hospital back in 2008. But for now, I can't see that happening when I have more patients to manage that I ever encountered as a medical student.

SURGERY IN WEST AFRICA

During my final year of medical school, my classmate and I had the opportunity to attend an international medical trip to Liberia, West Africa. Before leaving, I visited the Liberian Embassy in DC to obtain my visa and gain clearance into country. I also received vaccinations and collected prophylactic medications. I had never been to Africa before, and was excited about practicing Surgery and Emergency Medicine there.

We departed DC and flew to Paris, where we had a short, one hour layover – barely enough time to exit the plane and grab a quick bite from the airport restaurant. The airport was one of the largest I had ever visited. It was filled with hundreds of people, speaking foreign languages, and running in different directions to catch their flights. The food was *very* expensive, but I allowed myself to try some because I'd never had French food before. A slice of Quiche Lorraine and a fountain drink came to $21. Despite the amount it cost, I left feeling hungrier than before I had made the purchase because the portions were incredibly small. Still, I ignored my rumbling stomach and left to meet up with my colleague, Marci. Together, we boarded our plane.

Our plane was *enormous*! It was a double-deck plane with seats on both the lower level of the plane, where we sat, and upstairs. A single staircase led to the upper part of the plane. We then departed France and began the six-hour journey to John F. Kennedy (JFK) hospital in Monrovia, Liberia.

JFK was on the verge of recovery after the 1990s civil war that had devastated the country, including the hospital. Convicted war criminal and politician, Charles Taylor, had orchestrated the war. In the late 1980s, arbitrary rule and economic collapse culminated in civil war when Charles Taylor's National Patriotic

Front of Liberia (NPFL) militia seized and overran the country. Fighting intensified quickly, and approximately 250,000 people were killed while thousands more fled to neighboring countries. The conflict left the country in economic ruin, overrun with weapons and poverty, all of which was evident immediately upon entering the country.

As soon as we arrived in Liberia, I was anxious and excited to get off the plane and emerge into the African culture. The weather was muggy, but since the sun had already started going down, the temperature wasn't too unbearable. We made our way through customs without any problems and were greeted by Marci's family. They were waiting outside in a silver forerunner truck with Liberian license plates. As we loaded our bags into the truck, we were approached by two older males. One wasn't wearing any shoes. The other began making hand gestures, obviously suggesting he wanted some money. I was taken aback as the gentleman with no shoes attempted to open the door of the truck for me. I looked at Marci, and she looked just as confused as I was. The other gentleman didn't say a word. He just continued to make hand gestures to infer he wanted spare change. Apparently, opening doors for people (leaving and arriving) at the airport was an actual source of income for many people in Liberia. I searched my pockets and gave them both a few dollars. They graciously accepted my tip and then departed in the opposite direction.

We finished loading our bags into the truck, and then headed to the city of Monrovia. Despite the darkness outside, I was amazed at how many young children were walking the streets. Most of them were without shoes. The roads were poorly lit and filled with people walking while balancing food on their heads. Several kids played carelessly alongside them. Motorcycles swerved in and out of traffic as cars sped by, blowing their horns in excess. People were standing on the side of the road and selling everything from soap, underwear, scissors, gum, eggs, car fresheners, and carpet cleaner to firewood. Anything you needed, you could have found on those streets. People yelled through car windows at other cars that had broken down in the middle of the road. Other cars drove down the wrong side of the street to avoid waiting in traffic.

It was complete chaos!

My first thoughts were, *how close is the nearest hospital? Are there any ambulances around?* I was sure it wouldn't be long before I would witness an accident.

Our driver, Fiji, and I begin to have a conversation. I learned that he was also a medical student. The Liberian medical school takes five years to complete. The fifth year is for research and public health. It felt good to relate to someone, even though we were from two different cultures. We continued the treacherous path and finally made it to our destination – a house off the main road in a very small, secluded community. Chickens roosted while small children played outside with fire that was lit for trash and dirt. We stopped to have dinner and visit with Marci's relatives. We were served rice, plantains, corned beef, and fish. It was spicy, but delicious! This was followed by dessert and relaxation around the dinner table.

After dinner, we headed to the Methodist compound where we stayed for the month. After arriving, I grabbed my bags and headed towards the front door. I then noticed that there were no lights on in the house. Nonetheless, I grabbed a flashlight from my bag and headed inside. Apparently, the generator that provided electricity for the compound had broken down earlier in the day. And, even though it was late by the time we arrived, it was still very hot and muggy. The air conditioning had also stopped working when the generator went out. Luckily, there was a breeze from the Atlantic Ocean that could be felt throughout the house. When we listened closely, we could hear the waves through cracked windows, in the distance. Using my flashlight, I unpacked my bags and headed to the bathroom so I could shower, only to discover there was no running water.

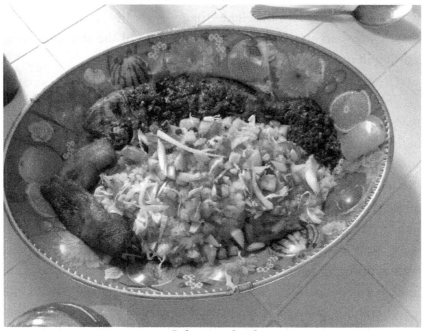

Liberian food

Thankfully, someone had ingeniously brought a large bucket of water into the house, taken from the nearby stream. With no running water, I was forced to improvise. I splashed the bucket of water onto my body, lathered up with soap, and used the remainder of the water to rinse. The realization began to sink in that I was in a third world country. I had to quickly remind myself why I was there.

Malaria is prevalent, not only in Liberia, but pretty much all throughout Africa. It is caused by a blood parasite, called *Plasmodium falciparum*, which is injected into humans when they are bit by mosquitos. To prevent this, we slept in bed nets so we wouldn't get bitten while asleep. We also brought prophylactic antibiotic medications to prevent contracting the deadly disease. I searched for my antibiotics, took two pills, and dozed off to sleep.

The next day, I got up extra early and put my freshly creased green scrubs on. I was eager to start working. I grabbed my stethoscope, threw it around my neck, and headed out the door. I arrived at the hospital and met with some of the General Surgery and Internal Medicine residents. We sat in a room, which also had no air conditioning, to receive report of patients that had come in the night before. Luckily, I found a face towel in my backpack and used it to wipe the sweat from my face throughout the report. After report, we met with the director of JFK Hospital, Dr. Long, and discussed what we wanted to gain from the rotation while in Liberia. I mentioned that I wanted to rotate in Surgery and also in the Emergency room. Marci stated the same. He was ok with that and was grateful just to have us come there to help at all.

After our meeting, we had a grand rounds lecture on Glaucoma by a Liberian Ophthalmologist. We learned that glaucoma is a devastating and often neglected problem in West Africa. It is the leading cause of blindness, second only to cataracts. Unfortunately, medications for its treatment are limited in Africa. Such a deficit in medication leads to permanent social economic and psychological disability. This lecture was followed by a discussion on healthcare in Liberia, which was moderated by several officials from the Health Ministry. Then, it was time to head to the operating room, where our first case was waiting.

The operating room was located on the 4th floor of the hospital. There was an elevator, but we didn't want to take the chance of it breaking down, so we took the stairs instead. The stairs were uneven and even broken in some spots. The lower step was short and small, and the upper step was wide and long. We had to watch our every step or risk tumbling down several flights of stairs. On the way up, I stopped and glanced at the surgical ward, which was located on the second floor. The floor was empty and quiet. Dirt and dust lined the concrete floors.

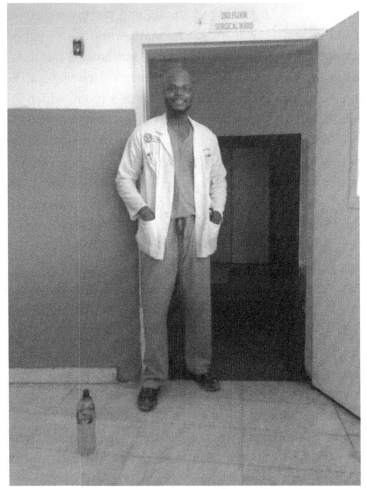

Outside the surgical floor

After what seemed like forever of walking up steps, we arrived on the 4th floor. The long hallways and empty rooms of the 4th floor painted the picture of a once deserted building ruined by the Liberian civil war. Wires hung from the ceiling, broken equipment collected in a corner pile, and the windows were cracked to let in the breeze from the Atlantic Ocean. The operating room windows actually overlooked the Atlantic Ocean. Close to the ocean was a small village, where young kids played in the dirt.

I immediately wondered why the kids were playing in the middle of the day and not at school.

Most of the surgical beds and instruments in the operating room had been donated to the hospital from other organizations. And this was very obvious, from how old and ancient the equipment was. Not only that, the lack of specialty physicians presented a larger problem. There was only one Orthopedic Surgeon in the country and he resided at JFK. There were no Urologists, no Cardiovascular Surgeons, no Neurologic Surgeons, no Plastic Surgeons, and no Anesthesiologists. A nurse, with additional training in airway and intubation, performed the anesthesia for our surgeries. I was taken by surprise when I learned that the nurse was using a drug, called Halothane, for the sedation of our patients. Halothane is rarely used in the US due to fatal complications to the liver and cardiac toxicity. Nonetheless, its cheap cost afforded the opportunity to sedate many patients over time, while keeping expenses low. Despite limited resources and manpower assistance, JFK hospital still managed to operate quite a bit.

Our first surgery was on a 42-year-old gentleman who had endured recurrent shoulder dislocations for the past two years. He was a manual laborer and his shoulder had gotten to a point where it prevented him from working. Our operation involved repairing the muscles and tendons around his shoulder to prevent further dislocations. The lack of supplies and equipment became more obvious midway through the case, when blood began to spurt from a nicked artery. To control bleeding during surgery in the US, there are cautery devices called bovies that are used to achieve hemostasis. After each case, the bovie tips are thrown away. In Liberia, that was not the case. There was one bovie tip and it was wiped off with betadine, after each surgery, to remove the prior patient's blood. This same bovie device was used on subsequent cases. All that mattered at that point though, was that we controlled and stopped the bleeding that had occurred as we cut into his shoulder.

After the case was completed, I left the operating room smiling from ear to ear. It felt like I had met a major milestone. That is, completing my first surgery in Africa, even if I was only the assistant.

Our next surgery was a thigh laceration debridement and repair. The patient was a 30-year-old, heavyset Liberian woman with long black hair. She was dressed in two hospital gowns, rigged together to keep her clothed and covered. She had a large laceration on her left inner thigh, which she reported happened three weeks prior, but refused to receive treatment for it at the time. It had started to become infected.

"Today, we will wash your leg and try to close your wound. Do you have any questions?" I asked her.

She nodded her head, inferring she didn't have any questions, and we took her back to the operating room.

In the US, when a patient has a wound that can't be closed with surgical sutures, we commonly place a device called a wound vac. This device is designed to decrease infection, assist in wound closure, and drain excess fluid. In Africa, there was no such thing. We improvised by internally rotating and maneuvering her leg to decrease tension so that we could close it. Miraculously, it worked and we were able to close her wound. I was thrilled because I was allowed to do some of the debridement and skin closure.

Our last case of the day was a 13-year-old female whose name was Edith. She had abdominal pain for one week prior to coming to the hospital. She appeared frightened as I examined her, but I tried to make her feel comfortable by sparking a conversation. There were no CT scanners, which we commonly use in the US when a patient presents with abdominal pain. There were no ultrasounds. We could, however, take her to surgery to cut open her belly. We needed to be sure that we thoroughly examined all of her abdominal and pelvic organs. A patient who presented with abdominal pain in Africa could have any number of diagnoses. One particular diagnosis that we were concerned about was Typhoid Fever. Another one was appendicitis. Typhoid Fever is endemic in Africa and is caused by a bacterium called *Salmonella.* It can lead to a number of symptoms. One particular symptom is abdominal pain, and can be fatal if missed.

We moved her back to the operating room and transferred her to the surgical table. When began the operation by making a large, 20 cm incision over the midline of her belly. As the surgeon started his incision on her belly, she began to move.

"The patient is moving!" yelled the head surgeon to the anesthesia nurse.

We waited several minutes until she was given additional paralytic medications. Then, we proceeded with the operation. We began the examination by first inspecting her small intestine. It appeared normal and without any areas of pathology. Then we examined her large intestine. It looked normal, except for a large collection of fluid near her appendix. Her appendix had ruptured and the fluid appeared to have been infected. This could have explained her abdominal pain. We were relieved that we found what was causing her to become so ill. If she would have waited any much longer, she likely would have became very sick and probably died. We removed her appendix, washed her belly with several liters of saline, and then sutured her belly closed. The next day, she went back home to be with her family and ultimately did well.

After the case, I looked over at my colleague. We both agreed that our first day was a success and decided to head home. We were thankful to be done with the day's cases, and grateful for the opportunity to help. We couldn't wait to come back the next day and perform more surgeries.

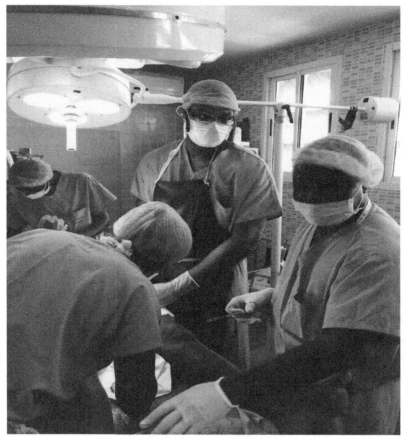

Operating room in Liberia

"YOU HAVE CANCER"

W e began the next day with a short lecture on malignant melanoma and filarial hydroceles, given by the surgery residents. Afterwards, we headed to clinic where multiple patients were lined up and waiting patiently outside on the benches. They stared as I walked up, and probably wondered what an American was doing at their hospital. I met up with the dean of the medical school, Dr. Bush, who was running late that day. He hurried in and headed straight for his desk.

Dr. Bush was an older Liberian doctor. He was dressed nicely in his crisp, white coat and polished, black dress shoes. He was known to push students academically, and expected a lot from them.

The clinic was a small room located near the front of the hospital. In it were two wooden desks, two plastic chairs, and an exam table. The only thing that separated the provider desks from the examining table was a makeshift wooden wall. This was used as a privacy barrier when patients got undressed for examinations. To cover the patients during exams, a white sheet was used. The very same sheet was used throughout the day on subsequent patients without being cleaned. There was also no sink to wash our hands in the clinic. Instead, we used hand sanitizer and had a bucket of water, which we poured over a trashcan to rinse our hands.

Our first patient was a 22-year-old male who had been seen in the clinic a few weeks prior. His name was Florian. He was told to return to clinic once he had his blood drawn. He was escorted to the clinic room by the nurse's aide and told to sit down near Dr. Bush.

"You have cancer," stated Dr. Bush.

Without taking the time to greet the patient or ask how he was doing, Dr. Bush gave him his diagnosis of cancer. Indeed, his test results and blood work pointed to the diagnosis of a liver tumor. The tumor was *large*! So large, in fact, that it had started causing his liver to fail. This was evident when I examined his eyes. They were yellow in color, a condition called jaundice. After learning he had cancer, Florian became mute as if he was shocked by what he had just heard. Thankfully, the patient's mom came along and spoke on his behalf.

"Are you saying there is nothing you can do for him?" she asked.

"Yes, unfortunately not. Come back to the clinic and see me in two months" Dr. Bush told her.

But we knew that likely wouldn't happen.

A big problem in Liberia was patient follow up and continuity of care. Most patients were told to return to clinic for follow up visits, but would never return. The ones who did return, returned too late. Their condition usually had progressed to irreversible and incurable states by that point.

Our next patient was a 45-year-old female who came in for a mass on her breast. She was dressed in a long black coat and wore dark sunglasses. I wondered why she was wearing a coat in the middle of the African summer. The nurse escorted her to the exam table, and I began my examination. As I lifted up her shirt, so that I could examine her breast, a strong pungent odor ran past my nose. I quickly glanced away. Throughout my years in the medical field and in the military, there were few things that I couldn't stomach. This was by far one of the worst I had ever seen. On her breast was a very large mass that appeared to be about 25-30 pounds. It was ulcerated, meaning it had been growing for some time. Other patients that were in clinic turned their nose in disgust as the odor quickly filled the room. She had wrapped the breast mass in a white shirt and had been carrying it around. She wore the long black coat for concealment. Like most other Liberian patients we were accustomed to seeing, she had delayed coming in to see a doctor. Instead, she went to a holistic doctor, then to church thinking prayer would work. Next, she went to cowboy doctors where they tried herbs and topical medications. The mass had continued to grow.

We needed to evaluate the extent of her breast cancer, so we ordered a chest X-ray. It confirmed our suspicion. The cancer had spread to her lungs and chest. There were no chemotherapy drugs in Liberia. There were no cancer doctors. There wasn't much more we could do for her. If she had presented sooner, we could have removed the tumor before it had spread. But, it was too late. We sent her home knowing that she would succumb to the breast cancer. I felt defeated and helpless at that point. I will never forget the look on her face when she left clinic that day.

After clinic we visited a Catholic school in Monrovia called, The Spiritan Academy. We went to speak to the kids about oral hygiene and healthy eating habits. We also showed them how to brush their teeth using large teeth models. They were very excited to see someone from America come and talk to them. It was especially gratifying to exchange jokes for smiles on their faces. During the talk, I found several kids giggling repetitively in the corner of the room. I joined them to see what was so funny. One of the students pointed at my lips, followed by several other students bursting out in laughs. Apparently, I have very pink lips — something uncommon in Africa where everyone is very dark.

Each kid at the school was required to wear a uniform to class. This consisted of brown khakis pants and a shirt with tie for the males. The girls wore green skirts with white shirts and bowties. The girls were also required to all have the same hairstyle — braids.

After I gave the talk, I remembered the patients we saw in clinic earlier that morning. The first patient had a liver tumor, but presented to clinic too late. Then, our patient with the breast mass hadn't bothered to see a doctor. Now she had an incurable breast cancer that had spread to her lungs. Whether that was from a lack of knowledge or just from personal traditional belief, both had waited too long.

I realized that a lot of the problems in Liberia revolved around the lack of public knowledge and education. A brilliant idea then popped into my head. What if we educated the school aged children about the common ailments and diseases that disproportionately affect Liberians? Then they could go home and teach their families. Such a thing could potentially dispel a lot of the misconceptions about medicine, and minimize delays in presentation.

That theory was short lived; as the bell rang indicating class was over. It may not have been the solution, but it was a good thought.

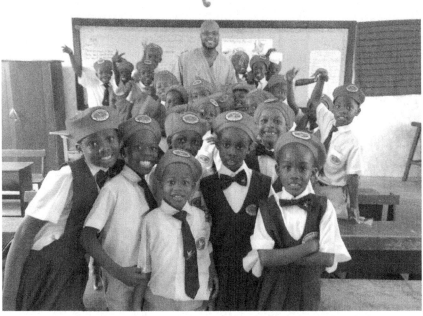

Spiritan Catholic Academy, Monrovia, Liberia 2014

GRATEFUL

The following day, we met with a local whose name was Lucian. He worked for an acquisitions company in Liberia, but was originally from Nigeria. Together, we ate burgers and fries at a restaurant called Golden Beach. We talked, relaxed, and enjoyed the nice scenery of the Atlantic Ocean. Before we knew it, it became dark. I had to work the day next day, so I said goodbye to everyone and started the walk home.

I had forgot my flashlight at the hospital, so I used my cell phone light instead. Since my arrival, I'd noticed streetlights on most of the streets, but I'd never seen any of them on. I kept my eyes on the ground to avoid tripping in a pothole or running into something along the street.

Out of nowhere a woman and two small kids appeared.

"I'm so sorry to bother you. Can I have a second of your time?" she asked.

I was somewhat skeptical, because it was late at night and dark outside. People walked aimlessly in the street and cars drove by without headlights on.

"Me and my children are very hungry. Can you help us get some food?" she asked.

I looked down at the little girl who stood beside her mother. She had big, bright eyes and her hair was pulled back in a ponytail. She was not wearing any shoes.

"Have you eaten today? I asked the little girl.

She shook her head and said, "No, we haven't eaten today."

"Why is that?" I asked.

"We don't have any money for food."

By that time, it was 9:00 pm, but I knew the temperature had risen to a scorching 110 degrees earlier in the day. I couldn't imagine going that long without food. Those small children hadn't eaten or probably even drank much water all day.

Luckily, there was a restaurant that served American food open across the street. I told her to follow me. Together, we walked to the restaurant and were met outside by two security guards. I noticed the guards had puzzled looks on their faces, so I didn't want to stir up a conversation. We quickly passed by them and headed inside the restaurant. Inside, every customer eating in the restaurant gave us the same confused look. They probably all wondered why there was an American in hospital scrubs with an older, poorly dressed lady in stained clothes with two young kids. The security guards, who were initially standing outside, appeared out of nowhere and began listening in on our conversation. To avoid making any more of a scene, I quickly gave a hand gesture to ensure them that there was no problem. I then grabbed a menu and handed it to the lady.

She handed it back.

"I want them to have Liberian food. That's all they eat," she stated.

I didn't want to cause any more commotion, so I gave in. By that time, the waitress started to look frustrated that we were taking up her time. To calm her down, I bought three bottles of water. I gave the lady and her kids the bottles of water and $10 in cash — all the money I had on me at the time.

"Here is my number. Call me if you all need anything," I told her.

Tears began to flow from her eyes. She then reached out for a big hug. I hugged her back and took one last look at her kids. I left the restaurant and headed home.

The entire way, I couldn't help but think about how unfair it was that people lived that way. They struggled day in and day out just to live, let alone eat. I could never imagine my children or family going for hours on end without food or water. I remembered back to the first day I arrived in country and how upset I was when the AC and water were out. I had to remind myself to continuously count my blessings and to *always* remain grateful.

…

The next morning, I was awakened by a loud honking sound from outside. I jumped up, grabbed my chocolate protein shake, and headed to the door to see who it was. It was our driver, Benjamin, who had come to pick us up and take us to another school to talk to some kids.

Benjamin was a tall, 50-year-old gentleman who had a head full of incoming grey hair. That day, he was wearing a brown button down shirt that he had neatly tucked into his trousers. We began to talk about Liberia and about how our lives were markedly different. He had been a driver for four years and told me he makes $80.00 a month. That seemed to be the common salary of most of the drivers in Liberia. I quickly added that amount up in my head and asked him again, to ensure that I heard him correctly.

"Yes, $80.00 a month", he said with a smile on his face.

I realized if he worked six days a week and roughly eight hours a day, his hourly rate would have been 38 cents an hour.

"It must be really hard to live off $80 a month?" I stated.

He nodded. He stated that he wanted to visit the US, but hasn't been able to because of poverty.

"The US looks beautiful. I've only seen pictures," he explained.

I tried to imagine living off such a small amount and quickly remembered that I had spent $90 the night prior, in less than five hours, on dinner.

That was his whole month's salary.

In the US, we often take things, such as fresh water, electricity, food, air conditioning, internet, and phones for granted. People in Liberia would do anything just to have a warm meal to eat or a place to call home. Since the war, cemeteries in Monrovia have become home for hundreds of people trying to find a place to live. They would remove the human remains or push the bones aside. Then, they slept on the tombs or sometimes inside them. Police raided the graveyards regularly and beat the people living there as they chased them away.

During my stay in Africa, our electricity worked 40% of the time. We went many days without running water or a working air conditioning. Many times, I found myself frustrated at the blazing heat and lack of fresh water, but I reminded myself that my stay there was temporary. I had the opportunity to return to a place where I never would have to worry about getting sick from drinking water, catching illnesses such as malaria, or trying to sleep in 90-degree heat without AC. On the other hand, this was the way of life for the Liberian people. But, they were very grateful for what they did have.

During these thoughts, I glanced back over at Benjamin. He was still wearing that same big smile, unchanged from 20 minutes ago.

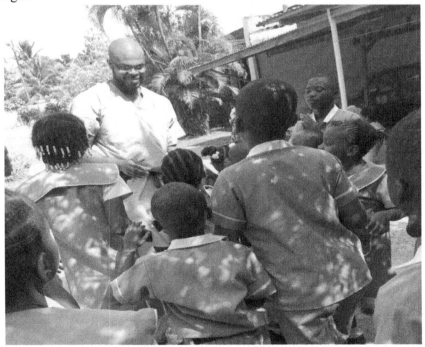

Speaking to students at a school in Paynesville, Liberia

EBOLA

In early June 2014, the city's first patient with Ebola arrived at Liberia's county hospital, Redemption. As tensions grew around the city of Monrovia, hospital administrators at JFK Hospital began to devise plans for handling patients with suspected Ebola.

Our grand rounds lecture the next day was given by officials from the Centers for Disease Control and Prevention (CDC). They came to Liberia to give us lectures about the deadly Ebola virus. They discussed prevention of spreading and what our plans would be in the event of a potential outbreak. Before that moment, there were no clear plans for what to do if a patient presented with symptoms of Ebola. No plans for isolation. No plans for treatment. To make matters worse, the scarcity of gowns, gloves, and personal protective attire presented a big problem.

At that point, we never imagined that Ebola would become so deadly and devastate a country so quickly.

After grand rounds, I headed down to the ER to meet with the head ER doctor. We met at the entrance of the ER. His name was Dr. Solomon and he was a black older gentleman dressed in an African dashiki shirt with light crisp blue pants. He immediately struck me as a very genuine person. He wore a large bright smile, along with dry weathered skin and thick brown eyeglasses. I soon learned that he was the father of six biologic and seven adopted children. He also trained in Germany in the early 70s. Despite the civil war that devastated the country, he returned to Liberia to work as an Emergency room physician, and to run his coffee plantation.

"Hi Dr. Solomon, I'm Antonio Webb, I'll be helping out today."

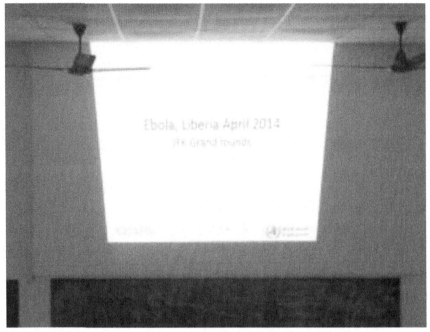

Our grand rounds lecture on Ebola from the CDC

"Ok great! Since you are here, I am going to head home and get some cashews."

He quickly left and headed out the ER back door.

My first patient was a 40-year-old diabetic female who came to the ER for a foot ulcer, likely from uncontrolled diabetes. The surgery team already had started antibiotics, but could not take her to the operating room because the schedule was full that day. I glanced down at her foot and then looked up at her. She was tearful and seemed embarrassed about waiting so long to come to the doctor. Her foot was mottled in appearance – she'd probably had the ulcer for some time. She had obviously waited until it started draining fluid and looked infected before she came in to be seen.

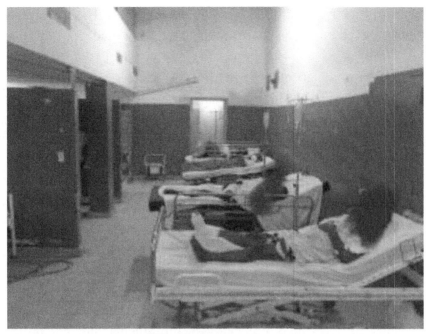

The Emergency Room

The nurse walked up to see what was going on.

"Can I get a pair of gloves please?" I asked.

She looked at me, rolled her eyes, and walked away. Ten minutes later, she returned with two gloves balled up in her scrub pocket. Even then, she hesitated about giving them to me.

Should I not be wearing gloves? Are we conserving them? I thought.

Nonetheless, I left to search for supplies to debride her foot. Supplies were limited, so I was forced to improvise and use whatever I could find. I found a surgical blade and pair of scissors, which were all the way on the other side of the ER.

Most patients with diabetes develop a condition called peripheral neuropathy, in which the high glucose levels damage small nerves that provide sensation to the foot. This creates a problem when patients bump their foot and then don't realize they have a wound, because they can't feel it. As I scraped away at her ulcer with a surgical blade, which I rigged onto a pair of scissors with tape, I realized that was the case. The lady's peripheral neuropathy was so bad that she didn't feel my blade as I cut into her skin.

"I am going to be honest with you and I want you to listen very carefully. Things like this can cause you to lose your foot. It is important that you take care of your health, eat right, and exercise," I told her.

She nodded her head and quickly looked away, as if she was embarrassed for letting her diabetes get out of hand.

Without time to even catch my breath, I overheard a nurse screaming to get my attention. A patient who was admitted the day prior with liver failure wasn't doing too well.

"Help, she's not breathing!" screamed the nurse.

I ran over to see what was going on. The patient's oxygen saturation was in the 60s (normal is 90-100%). Her breathing was irregular, often a sign of impending death, called agonal breathing.

I checked her heart rate and could not feel one. She was essentially dead at that point.

"Start CPR," I yelled.

The respiratory therapist climbed on top of the bed and immediately started pumping on her chest.

I ordered the nurse to give 1mg of epinephrine and instructed another nurse to grab the defibrillator. I rechecked her heart rate and still felt nothing. By that time, the respiratory therapist was drenched in sweat from doing CPR. The hospital had no AC, and I was told to hydrate at every chance. Everywhere I went inside the hospital, I carried a fresh bottle of water to avoid drinking the Liberian water.

We stopped CPR to check her rhythm on the monitor: Ventricular fibrillation (V-fib).

V-fib occurs when the heart does not pump properly and just quivers. It's a life threatening arrhythmia and an indication for defibrillation. I grabbed the two defibrillator paddles and told everyone to stand clear. I then shocked her with 200 joules of electricity. When she jumped from the electricity of the defibrillator, I jumped as well, startled. Even though I saw it during medical school, I never had to shock a patient back to life myself and had never run a code blue alone.

I glanced over at the monitor. Flat line_____

At that point, I knew what we were doing was futile. Had the patient survived the cardiac arrest, she would likely have died from liver failure. In addition, the hospital was devoid of Lactulose, a medication given to patients with hepatic encephalopathy.

Even though she had flat lined, and I knew it wasn't indicated, I wanted to shock her again. *What would we lose?* I thought.

This time, I used 300 joules of electricity. She jumped. Still nothing.

The flat line remained_____

Even after everything we had done, nothing would bring her back.

Time of death: 10:15am.

Minutes later, an older gentleman with a history of a heart condition, called atrial fibrillation, came in with right-sided weakness and slurred speech. Instinct told me he had likely had an embolic stroke from his heart condition. He admitted to taking his aspirin that morning, but may have not been taking it regularly.

We learn in medical school that, 'time is muscle.' All we had at that point, however, was time. In the US, we send suspected stroke patients immediately to the CAT scanner and activate a stroke team. Then, we administer medications to restore blood flow to the brain.

There was no such thing in Liberia. No stroke team. No CAT scan machines. No medication for strokes. Just time.

And time we were wasting.

He sat on the ER stretcher and stared at the ceiling walls. We could not do anything for him. He had most likely suffered continuous brain damage. This left him with permanent and irreversible neurological and social economic damage, something that is very much preventable in the US.

While I attempted to gather the rest of his history, a nurse ran over to tell me her patient wasn't doing well.

Her patient was a 33-year-old female who had delivered a baby vaginally, a few days ago in a back alley. Now she had shortness of breath and signs of a blood infection. I instructed the nurse to give her a 500ml bolus of fluid, even though her urine output had been low and her blood creatinine levels were high: signs that her kidneys were failing. The nurse quickly gave her the fluids. It didn't affect her blood pressure much and instead her oxygen saturation dropped. I glanced over at my colleague, who had just arrived, and we gave each other the same nervous, "I don't know what to do" look.

"We have to make a decision – now! Otherwise, she will die," my colleague said.

I ordered the respiratory therapist to gather supplies so we could intubate her. Before that point, I had only intubated patients under the supervision of anesthesiologists in the operating room, on my anesthesia rotation in medical school. But, there was no time to ponder. We needed to act fast!

The respiratory technician returned and handed me an endotracheal tube, which looked like it had been used.

"I need a new tube," I quickly stated.

"We wash our endotracheal tubes and re-use them," he responded.

Even though I was in disbelief by what I had just heard, I didn't have time to put up a fight. Our patient was crashing – and crashing fast!

We decided that Marci, my colleague, was to intubate while I tried to insert a tube in her nose to decompress her belly. Her belly seemed to be swelling by the minute. As Marci inserted her breathing tube, the patient began to vomit. We suctioned the regurgitated fluid and turned her on her left side. Her oxygen saturation was now in the 80s and her blood pressure dropped to 40/20.

She was crashing!

I glanced over at the monitor and noticed that her heart rate was *zero* on the monitor. I felt for a pulse. There was none. Without hesitating, I started pumping on her chest as hard as I could, even after hearing her ribs crack between my fingers. I instructed the nurse to retrieve the defibrillator from the other side of the ER. I prepared the paddles with lubrication and stopped CPR to check her heart rhythm. Thankfully, her heart was beating again, but unorganized — a condition known as ventricular tachycardia. I placed the paddles on her chest, and shocked her with 200 joules of electricity.

"Give her another milligram of epinephrine," I yelled out to a nurse who was just standing back and looking on. She appeared to be startled by everything that was going on.

I rechecked the patient's pulse, which was much stronger now. It was possible that adrenaline we just pushed into her veins had caused her heart rate to increase. Her oxygen saturation slowly dwindled back up. And, then her eyes opened.

Whew! We saved her life. She was in critical condition, but stable.

Did we do everything right? Did we miss something? I thought.

Sure, she had a blood infection. She had warm skin, low blood pressure, a high heart rate, fever of 102.7, and low urine output – all of which pointed to a diagnosis of sepsis. But, was there anything we could have done differently? There were none of the medications we commonly give in the US when a patient doesn't respond to initial intravenous fluids. Instead, we improvised by injecting 1ml of adrenaline into a bag of 500ml saline and then used that to raise her blood pressure back up to normal range. In medical school, we learn that the mortality for someone who goes into cardiac arrest is very high. However, all that mattered at that point was that we saved her life.

I sat down to catch my breath, my mind running through everything that had occurred during the day. *The day had been insane!* One of my patients died. Another patient was at risk for losing her foot. Another patient had a stroke and there was nothing we could do for him. And, I almost lost another patient.

I never would have imagined that I would be numb and desensitized to the loss of a patient. Maybe it was the adrenaline that had been flowing in my veins since my arrival in the ER that morning. Maybe it was from serving in war and all the gruesome injuries and deaths I witnessed. Maybe it was because the ER had been so busy that day, and there was no time to mourn. Maybe it was because I had never been in a situation where I had to make decisions that would ultimately save or end a patients' life. That day, I had to make those decisions. And, even though I made the appropriate decisions, my patient still passed.

Being a physician involves treating patients and showing compassion and empathy. It also involves going home and acting normal, separating all feelings from the day. Most physicians learn to do this over time after years of practice; I guess I learned it a lot sooner.

It was only then that I remembered the ER doctor who left earlier in the morning to get cashews. He never came back. As soon as he had left, things started going downhill. I shook my head and thought to myself, "Welcome to Africa!"

I soon left Liberia and was fortunate to not contract Ebola, although I treated several patients with suspected symptoms. Unfortunately, I cannot say the same for everyone that I worked with while there. A few weeks after my departure, Ebola became rampant in Liberia. It further weakened and destroyed a country that was already on the verge of recovery from the 1990's civil war, led by militant Charles Taylor.

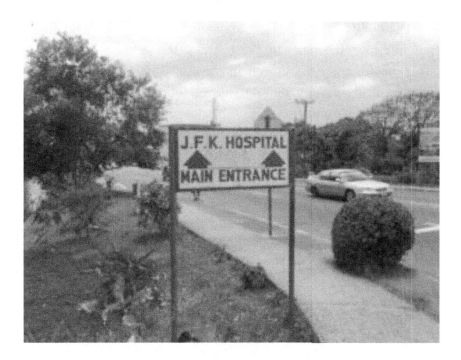

The virus soon spread to neighboring countries, Sierra Leone and Guinea. As of October 2014, the World Health Organization (WHO) and the Centers for Disease Control and Prevention (CDC) have reported more than 8,000 suspected cases and more than 3,000 confirmed deaths.

The Liberian medical infrastructure was not ready for such a deadly outbreak. The WHO estimated that Liberia's capacity for treating Ebola was insufficient by over 2,000 beds. In some areas of Liberia, protestors began attacking hospitals because they thought the disease was a hoax and the hospitals were responsible for the disease. Many areas of Liberia that were seriously affected by the virus lacked basic supplies and had limited access to soap and clean, running water.

The virus soon took the life of Dr. Solomon, Dr. Long, and several other physicians that I worked with while there. JFK Hospital closed its doors to patients not much longer after, eliminating what minimal healthcare that had existed.

The WHO later released a statement that said, "The Ebola epidemic ravaging parts of West Africa is the most severe acute public health emergency seen in modern times. Never before in recorded history has a biosafety level four pathogen infected so many people so quickly, over a broad geographical area, for so long."

Rest in peace to the doctors I met while there. They placed their lives on the line and passed away doing something they enjoyed doing — helping others. They cared for patients, despite inadequate and unsafe resources, clean water, air conditioning, supplies, and insufficient training in infection control. These selfless doctors were on the front lines, and died as a result. They continued to sacrifice themselves to provide for others, even after a deadly disease such as Ebola wreaked havoc throughout their country.

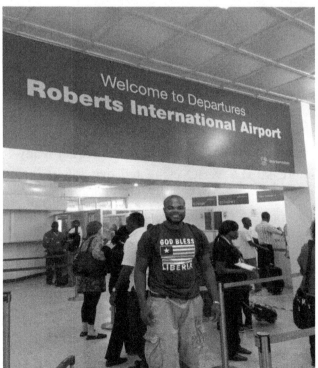

GOD BLESS LIBERIA!

BE DIFFERENT

Everything I've achieved in life, I earned. From buying my first house at the age of 22, to working my way through college, to financing my way through medical school for my Doctorate of Medicine (M.D.), I earned it. I went from the rough streets of Louisiana to the streets of Boston at Harvard. The majority of my colleagues have parents, brothers, sisters, aunts, and uncles who are physicians. And the list goes on. For these individuals, success and matriculation comes naturally. They are constantly fed information on success, what preparation courses to take, and what next step to take to achieve a particular goal. Nonetheless, I am grateful and blessed for the opportunity and for the struggle. Fredrick Douglass said it best when he said, "Without struggle, there is no progress." If my parents had given me everything, I would not be the person I am today. I would not be as hungry, as humble, or as fortunate as I am today.

Seeing my father struggle day in and day out ignited a spark in me early in life, which has yet to be put out. Growing up around drugs, gangs, and violence tends to create a vicious cycle where it seems like there is no way out. Generations after generations repeat this process, often losing family members along the way to drugs, prison, or a grave six feet under. Poverty further complicates this. My goal is to break this cycle of poverty of living below one's means, and from paycheck-to-paycheck.

Imagine that you were the only person living on this earth. Ask yourself, would you still buy those $4,500 rims? Would you still buy those $300 Jordan shoes? Would you still spend $1,000 on a bottle of liquor at the club? Most people spend excessive amounts of money because they see everyone else doing it. They spend money to "Keep up with the Joneses." This philosophy has widespread effects on our society and on our thought process. According to this philosophy, conspicuous consumption occurs when people care about their standard of living in relation to their peers. We live in a very superficial society. This influences our decision making process when it comes to making purchases and everyday decisions.

I've spent and wasted thousands of dollars over the years on car rims, stereo systems, and expensive paint jobs. Looking back, I have nothing to show for it. Yes, we live and we learn but the sooner you learn and recognize this, the wealthier you will become. That $15,000 I spent over the years could easily be $50,000 or more today. That's if I would have invested it wisely.

Moral of the story: Be different. Don't follow the crowd.
The majority of people who you see with nice $75,000 cars and $1,000,000 homes are broke. In one of my favorite books, *The Millionaire Next Door*, author Thomas Stanley mentions that most millionaires aren't who you think they are. Most millionaires act, think, and live frugal. They drive older cars (which they saved and paid for with cash) and live in appropriately sized homes (which are paid off).

If you want to be rich, you need to stop acting like you have money in the bank and start living beneath your means. Motivational Speaker and Financial Author Dave Ramsey once said, "If you will live like no one else, later you can live like no one else."

As I went off to medical school, the demographics quickly changed. I suddenly found myself around very intelligent people who didn't talk about how big their rims were or how much they paid for the candy paint on their car. Instead, I heard conversations about stocks, bonds, politics, and who the next president would be. Two completely different worlds. What I had imagined would be most difficult, was actually an easy transition. Instead of being around the typical Louisiana native whose dialect may have been hard to understand, while at Georgetown, I found myself around individuals who spoke eloquently.

I quickly realized that I needed to change my ways in order to fit in. Growing up, I often spoke fast. Speaking rapidly, combined with my Louisiana dialect, made it difficult for people to understand my conversation. Many times, at Georgetown, I would often hear big words that I didn't understand or had never heard of. I went home and searched those words online and started incorporating them into my vernacular. There is an old adage that says, "If you hang out with chickens, you're going to cluck and if you hang out with eagles, you're going to fly." After being around my colleagues at Georgetown, I wanted to be like them by speaking intelligently and ranting off political verbiage unapologetically. I wanted to be among the eagles and fly. Don't get me wrong, there is nothing wrong with people in Louisiana. Louisiana is my home. But, to be successful you have to be different. I wanted to be different from those I grew up with. When I go back to Shreveport these days, I see the same people I grew up with doing the same things they were doing when I left Shreveport in 2001. They are stuck in a repetitive cycle.

This is not the case for everyone. There have been many successful people who have come out of Shreveport, and many wealthy people who currently reside in Shreveport who do a lot of great things for the city.

I also changed the way I dressed when I arrived at Georgetown. While out one day with friends at a local bar, the bouncer asked, after checking my ID, "Why is your shirt so big?" I didn't know what he meant at that time, but thinking back, I now realize what he meant. I looked ridiculous wearing 4XL shirts, which came to almost my knees, and pants so big that my imaginary twin could also have fit inside them. That was the norm in Louisiana – baggy clothes. At Georgetown, it was just the opposite. Everyone dressed preppy and I liked that about being there. I slowly threw out all my oversized clothes and began dressing the part.

ADVICE:

You have to be a chameleon in life. Flexible. Adaptable. You will go in and out of various environments and will be faced with challenges in all of them. As a minority or African American, people will expect you to be inferior or to not know as much as others. I made it my goal to circumvent this during medical school by studying harder, reading longer, and partying less. Don't get me wrong, I did party, but I often cut it short to hit the books a little longer than my colleagues. You have to be prepared to have a conversation with your boy from the hood, and minutes later have an intelligent conversation with the Vice President of the hospital. It takes lots of practice, but is very possible. How I speak to my patients at the hospital or my surgery colleagues is completely different from how I would speak to my boys back home. It's a very important and valuable learned trait.

BONUS: FIVE PEARLS FOR SUCCESS

1. *Put God First*

Proverbs 3:6 says, "In everything you do, put God first and he will direct you and crown your efforts with success." There are so many things that clamor for our attention such as our job, kids, family, sports – the normal demands and distractions of life. No one is perfect, as we all have fallen short of the glory of God. We have to be careful and not let these things distract us from our relationship with God. Matthew 6:31-33 states, "Therefore do not be anxious, saying, what we shall eat? What shall we drink? What shall we wear? For the Gentiles seek after all these things, and your heavenly father knows that you need them all. But seek first the kingdom of God and his righteousness, and all these things will be added to you."

I, myself, find this hard to do at times. We get so caught up in our daily routines of school, work, and family that we tend to neglect the person who actually blessed us with a roof over our head, clothes on our back, and food on our table. The key to having God's abundant life is to keep him in our priorities. When you decide to serve God with your whole heart and make him first in your life, your soul will prosper and your joy and peace will increase.

2. *Invest in yourself:*

In an ABC news interview in July of 2009, when asked whether it is still important for families to send their children to college or higher learning, Warren Buffett stated, "Generally speaking, investing in yourself is the best thing you can do. Anything that improves your own talents, nobody can tax it or take it away from you. They can run up huge deficits and the dollar can become worth far less. You can have all kinds of things happen. But if you've got talent yourself, and you've maximized your talent, you've got a tremendous asset that can return ten-fold."

Instead of buying that next set of 26" rims or that car stereo player (both of which when you look back ten years from now, you will wonder what happened to that item or money), invest in yourself. Learn a new language such as Spanish or French; improve your communication skills; get braces and whiten your teeth; join a local gym; buy and read books on investing health, or fitness; or take piano lessons to create new brain circuitry. Learning a new language is a valuable tool in your arsenal of success. The military and other employers will actually pay you extra money if you speak a second language. And, it's a great feeling to be the only person who can translate a conversation for others.

An independent research firm, Kelton Research, found that your smile might also land you your next dream job. They found that applicants are 58% more likely to get a job offer and 53% more likely to be offered an increased salary if their teeth were white and straight. It was an easy decision for me to correct the alignment of my teeth by spending $4,500 on Invisalign. Your teeth are one of the first things people notice about you, and it's something you can look back on 20 years later and know exactly where that $4,500 went. These are the kind of investments and purchases that you want to make.

3. *Surround yourself with like-minded, sound people*

Like I mentioned previously, you are whom you hang around and associate with. When I return home to Louisiana to visit my family, the majority of my childhood friends are doing the same thing as when I left over ten years ago — sitting on the block, rolling dice, smoking weed, and most of them still living with their parents. As I have become older, I have become more strict and vigilant about who comes around me and who I associate with. The majority of my close friends are successful and are surgeons, businessmen/businesswomen, lawyers, engineers, and investors. These are the type of people you want to associate with. Use them to your advantage. Challenge them. Be inquisitive. Ask lots of questions. Take them to dinner and pick their brains. Otherwise what is the point of having them around? If you know someone who makes a lot of money from the stock market, invite him or her to dinner and pick his or her brain the entire time. That $20 you spent on the dinner could help make you thousands or millions of dollars later.

I first started investing in stocks when I was in medical school. I was really busy with schoolwork and didn't really have the time to sit down and read about how to set limits, buy, sell, trade, etc. I ended up losing $800 on a sale and decided to take a break from it to focus on studying. A good friend of my family is a day trader and buys and sells thousands of dollars' worth of stock every day. I invited him out to dinner one evening. He was not aware of my intentions. During dinner, I essentially asked him hundreds of questions about investing, which stocks were the best ones to buy, which brokerage company he uses, etc. He explained to me what he does and how he makes thousands of dollars a week from buying and selling stock. I was learning so much that I didn't even get a chance to enjoy my meal. I was ecstatic and ran home that night to buy several e-books on investing to reinforce what I had learned.

After completion of medical school, I decided to start investing again. One morning after a long night of work, I decided to buy stock in a restaurant called El Pollo Loco. They had just made a public offering a few days prior. My best friend said, "We need to buy some El Pollo Loco stock, it's going to sky rocket." I kind of brushed him off and said I would look into it. He ended up buying 125 shares at $19/share. I woke up to a text message from him saying his account had grown over $1,000 in just a few hours.

I was envious and wanted in. The next day, I decided to invest and bought 30 shares, spending about $600. I went to sleep and woke up several hours later to check the stock market. I had made $250. The best thing about it was that I made it while asleep and didn't use any energy to earn it. The only thing I used was glucose for brain metabolism while asleep. At that point, I was hooked and was ready to read more about investing and stocks.

Set yourself up for financial success by making your money work for you. So even if you are at home in bed, wearing a gown and slippers, your money is still working for you.

My best friend and I have been friends since attending Hollywood Middle School in Shreveport, Louisiana. We then attended Southwood High School. He was the class president and valedictorian of our class. We both graduated with honors. When everyone else was running the streets and hitting on females, we were hitting the books. Our friends used to make fun of us for studying so much, and because we headed inside early at night to prepare for upcoming exams. Looking back now, neither of us have any regrets. We are both very successful because of the sacrifices we made while younger. He is a Duke trained Cardiothoracic Anesthesiologist, and I am an Orthopedic Surgeon in residency. During high school, he approached me one day and said, "Let's apply for some scholarships and go to college together." We were both excited to finish high school and to get out of Shreveport, but my plans were to gain medical experience before applying to medical school. He applied and was granted several college scholarships. He chose to attend Xavier University for college and went straight to LSU for medical school afterwards. I, conversely, decided to go into the military so that I could have a way to pay for college and also gain medical experience. I have no regrets in the path I took, albeit it took me five years longer to obtain my Doctorate of Medicine degree. Someone once said, "The path to our destination is not always a straight one. We go down the wrong road, we get lost, and we turn back. Maybe it doesn't matter which road we embark on. Maybe what matters is that we embark." Even though I didn't go the traditional route of high school to college, and from college to medical school, in the end I still achieved my goal of becoming a doctor.

Don't base your goals or decisions on what the next person is doing. Set a goal and accomplish it, regardless of everyone else's plans. It may not be the easiest goal to obtain, and you should know that there will be blocks and bumps along the way. Take these obstacles and learn from them, as I did during my journey of becoming a doctor. My best friend and I are set to become millionaires in the next few years due to the hard work and sacrifices we made while we were younger. What can you do today that will set you up for success in the future?

4. *Watch less TV, listen to less music, and read more:*

I cannot stress enough how many hours of your day and life are wasted away watching gossip and reality TV. Think about it. Say for instance you spend only two hours a day watching TV, which is totally underestimated. The New York Daily Times reported that an average American spends 34 hours a week watching TV. Times that by six months and you will have wasted over 300 hours of your life watching TV and gained nothing positive from it. Research has shown that when you are watching TV, your higher brain regions shut down and activities shift to the lower brain regions. The lower portion of your brain is set in a "fight or flight" response mode while your higher brain regions undergo atrophy due to lack of usage. Numerous studies have also shown that TV viewing among children leads to lower attention and poorer brain development.

Instead, replace those one or two hours of TV with a good book or podcasts (which are free apps to download). I actually don't have cable and rarely watch TV, except for sporting events and special occasions. In addition, I rarely listen to music. Most music and rappers these days talk about drugs, money, cars, and sex. What are you learning and taking away from listening to that type of music? Instead, listen to Dave Ramsey (financial guru), Joel Osteen (mega church pastor), or Bill Gunderson (stock investor guru). Just imagine how much more knowledgeable you will be if you cut out music for an entire year and listened to "Spanish Made Easy" or "Investing in Stocks 101." I'm not saying that you should cut out all music. Music is therapeutic and a stress reliever. I listen to it religiously while working out. Listen to it, but don't let it consume all your time. Just imagine how much you would know about stocks, bonds, and investing if you didn't listen to music while driving. Instead, listen to experts and millionaires talk about how they became successful by buying and selling stocks and real estate.

A study in 2011 showed that Americans spend, on average, more than a full workweek in traffic. Washington, DC is notorious for having bad and congested traffic. DC is arguably the most congested urban city in the US, followed by Los Angeles, San Francisco, New York, and Boston. In medical school, I used this to my advantage while coming home from class or from clinical rotations. While waiting in traffic, I listened to audio lectures and played podcasts. Imagine if you could take that full workweek of sitting in traffic and learn about real estate. You will become very knowledgeable in the real estate market in no time.

5. *Apply the 3 D's of success to your life: Discipline, Determination and Dedication:*

The discipline to stay focused, determination to keep going, and the dedication to never give up. My greatest memory and lesson learned from the military is the discipline that was bestowed upon my fellow troops and I. This would ultimately set me up for success in medical school and allow me to match into one of the most competitive specialties in medicine. My militaristic style study regimen consisted of, on average, 12-16 hours of study each day. My classmates and friends often envied me because of this and often sought after me for advice. I ended up becoming a highly requested tutor to medical students, and helped them develop effective and structured study plans. The nights that I did end up going out to hang with friends, I made sure to get back home at a reasonable time to be up bright and early the next morning to begin studying again. A day missed of studying in medical school is like missing two weeks of college work, so it was wise not to get behind.

Whatever career you decide to enter and whatever goal you set for yourself, think of it as a marathon and not a race. When I volunteered to run a 5K race in medical school for a community fundraiser, I knew I was out of shape the moment we first started running. I knew that in order for me to make it to the finish line, I needed to pace myself. Those quick long strides that first propelled me from the starting line quickly turned into rhythmic and coordinated slower paced strides. Even though individuals twice my age reached the finish line several minutes before me, I successfully completed the 5K race because I paced myself.

Success cannot be rushed and does not come overnight. It requires determination and the will power to keep going mentally when your body is physically telling you to quit. Trust me, you will be faced with obstacles over and over in life and you will want to quit. Don't give up, no matter what. Keep that coordinated stride towards the finish line and don't look back.

You must also have the dedication to devote yourself completely with both your heart and mind. Vince Lombardi once said, "The price of success is hard work, dedication to the job at hand, and the determination that whether we win or lose, we have applied the best of ourselves to the task at hand." Having the dedication to stick with your goals in the face of obstacles and setbacks will become vital as you go through life. You will want to quit, but don't!

Lastly, stay true to yourself. Work hard and continue reaching toward your goals in life, even when you are faced with failure or met with the challenge of "Overcoming the Odds."

ACKNOWLEDGEMENTS

First, I would like to thank God for blessing me with the knowledge, vision, and patience to write this book. Without him, none of this would have been possible. I also would not be at the point where I'm at in life. According to the statistics, I should be dead or in jail but because of his mercy, I am able to inspire and motivate others to follow my path to success instead of a path which leads to prison or six feet under. To my beloved brother, Jonathan Immanuel Webb, who motivated and inspired me by his intelligence and by his love for computers. Rest in peace. I miss you dearly. My pops, John Webb: I am the person today because of you. You could have been like many other fathers I knew so well growing up and left us to be raised by foster parents or other family members. Instead, you made it a point to keep us together and did everything you could to make that happen. My mother, Yvette Webb, who has endured a lot over the years, overcame an addition with drugs and who I am proud of. I love you mom! My older brother, Chris Webb, who has been a role model to me over the years and taught me about life, real estate, finance, investing, and entrepreneurship. More importantly, my relationship with God has become stronger because of watching yours. Thank you for everything. To my sister Nicole, I am proud of you. You are very beautiful and smart. I am blessed to call you my sister. To my stepmother, Teresa Webb, thank you for everything over the years.

A special thanks to Dr. Lita Powell who spent countless hours helping me edit and put together this book. I love you!

There are too many people, outside my immediate family, to mention but just know that I really appreciate all of you for the support!

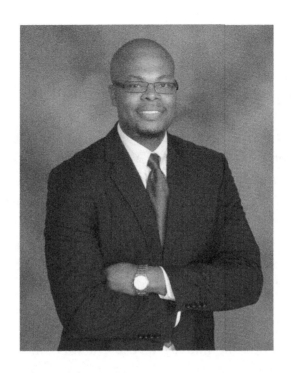

ABOUT THE AUTHOR

The odds were stacked against Antonio Webb, beginning with his childhood in Shreveport, Louisiana. Friends and family members were serving jail time, or addicted to drugs. Some close friends were even killed amidst the challenges of the neighborhood.

With these influences in his life, it seemed he was destined to turn out the same way. But fate had something else in mind for young Webb. While in high school, he developed an interest in biology and medicine and his grades earned him a spot in a local medical magnet program for disadvantaged students. Inspired by this experience, he began to dream of a career as a doctor, even though no one in his immediate family had completed college, let alone medical school.

Webb realized his best chance for financial help with higher education would come if he served in the military. After 17-year-old Webb graduated high school in the top 5% of his class, his father consented to let him join the U.S. Air Force, in 2001.

While on his 8-year active duty commitment in the Air Force, Webb worked as a medic and simultaneously attended undergrad at the University of Texas at San Antonio, taking classes whenever and wherever he could to compete his degree. 6 1/2 years after first beginning, Webb became the first person in his family to hold a college degree.

He was later deployed north of Baghdad, Iraq, where he served as a combat medic; on a base dubbed "Mortarville" for the frequency of mortar attacks it endured. He treated just over 800 patients during his deployment and earned several medals in the process.

When he left the military in 2009, it was time to pursue his medical training full time, beginning with the Georgetown Experimental Medical Studies Program, which worked to prepare students from disadvantaged backgrounds for success in medical school and beyond. From there, he was accepted into the renowned Georgetown University School of Medicine, and he says he considers the day he was accepted the most unforgettable moment of his life thus far.

His studies covered medicine as well as medical research and he earned honors in the fields of Renal, Pediatrics, Internal Medicine, Surgery, Psychiatry and Critical Care ICU, leading to his Doctorate of Medicine degree in 2014.

Today, Dr. Antonio Webb is completing his residency at the University of Texas, San Antonio in Orthopedic Surgery with plans to specialize in Trauma Orthopedic Surgery.

During his free time, he loves serving as a mentor for underprivileged middle and high school students interested in a career in medicine. He volunteers to help because he says it is important for students to know "If I can do it, they can, too." Webb

210

says his proudest moment would be when he encounters a student in later years who says, "I am in medical school because of you."

It's been a long road from impoverished child in a dangerous environment to decorated soldier and award-winning medic, and Antonio Webb, MD is aware of the amazing journey that has been his life. "I don't take anything for granted," he says. "I know I am incredibly blessed."

SPEAKING ENGAGEMENTS

Teachers, Counselors, Program directors, Youth Ministers, Professors, Corrections Officers….. Book Dr. Webb to come speak at your event!

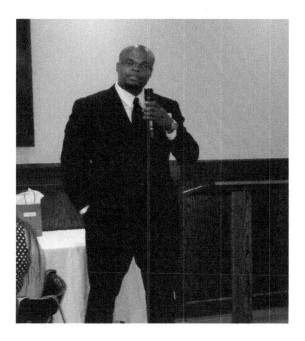

You can expect to receive from me:
1. Timely and prompt phone call and email returns
2. A 45 minute-1hour engaging speaking event that is tailored to your club, program or organization.
3. Book signing and picture taking at the end of the event
4. Publicity: The event will be promoted on my social media sites to thousands of my followers.

Contact:
overcomingtheoddsbook@gmail.com

FROM THE AUTHOR

Thank you for the support. I truly appreciate it!

All I ask is that after you read this book, bless someone else with it.

I would love to hear from you. Email:
overcomingtheoddsbook@gmail.com
-
or connect with me at:
-
www.antoniowebbmd.com
www.twitter.com/drwebb82
www.youtube.com/antoniowebbmd
www.facebook.com/awebbmd
www.linkedin.com/in/antoniowebbmd
www.amazon.com/author/antoniowebbmd
www.instagram.com/overcomingtheoddsbook

BIBLIOGRAPHY

"1 in 3 black males will go to prison in their lifetime" web sept 14
http://www.huffingtonpost.com/2013/10/04/racial-disparities-criminal-justice_n_4045144.html

"Shreveport-Bossier ranked 12th most dangerous metro area in country." Web June 13.
http://www.ksla.com/story/2602240/shreveport-bossier-ranked-12th-most-dangerous-metro-area-in-country

"The importance of fathers in the healthy development of children." Web Oct 13
https://www.childwelfare.gov/pubs/usermanuals/fatherhood/chaptertwo.cfm.com

"Ten ways to be a great dad" web Sept 14
http://www.nyc.gov/html/hra/nycdads/html/campaign/10_ways.shtml.com

"What college degrees produce the most millionaires?" web July 14.
http://education.yahoo.net/articles/majors_popular_with_millionaires.htm

Collins, S. Emergency Medical Support Units to Critical Care transport teams in Iraq. Crit Care Nurse Clin N Am 20 (2008) 1-11

"Understanding the five branches of the military," Nov 14
http://www.militaryspot.com/enlist/understanding-the-five-branches-of-the-military/

"Mass casualty and military triage web Sept 14
http://www.cs.amedd.army.mil/borden/FileDownloadpublic.aspx?
docid=68aca9a0-9cd7-4d8f-a17f-a4c01264daef

"Recognizing the signs of PTSD" web June 14.
http://www.psychologytoday.com/blog/workings-well-
being/201307/recognizing-the-signs-post-traumatic-stress.com

"Choosing a major or career path" web Sept 14
http://careercenter.depaul.edu/advice/majorcareerpath.aspx

"8 College degrees that will earn your money back" web Sept 14
www.salary.com/8-college-degrees-that-will-earn-your-money-
back/.com

"Criminal records and background checks affect Employment at
DMV. Web July 14
http://www.dmv.org/articles/how-criminal-records-affect-
employment.com

"Centers for disease control and prevention, High blood pressure"
web Sept 13
http://www.cdc.gov/bloodpressure/.com

"The types of Schizophrenia" Web June 13
http://www.mentalhealthamerica.net/conditions/schizophrenia.com

"5 reasons why you should commit your goals." Web Oct 13
http://michaelhyatt.com/5-reasons-why-you-should-commit-your-
goals-to-writing.html

"5 things successful people do that others don't." Web Sept 14 https://www.americanexpress.com/us/small-business/openforum/articles/5-things-successful-people-do-that-others-dont/

Chen D, Lew R, Hershman W. (2007). A cross-sectional measurement of medical student empathy. *J Gen Intern Med., (10): 1434-8*

"10 things that Michael Jordan can teach you about facing failure in your writing career." Web Sept 14
http://justwritedamnit.com/10-things-michael-jordan-can-teach-facing-failures-writing-career/

Mugele, Josh. A Good Death. The New England Journal of Medicine, September 3, 2014DOI: 10.1056/NEJMp1410301

"U.S. commuters on average spend nearly a week stuck in traffic." Web Sept 13
http://www.reuters.com/article/2013/02/05/us-usa-transportation-congestion-idUSBRE91406X20130205